# Dental Emergencies

# Dental Emergencies

## Edited by

## Mark Greenwood
MDS, PhD, FDS, FRCS, FRCS (OMFS), FHEA

*Consultant and Honorary Clinical Professor*
*Newcastle University*

## Ian Corbett
BDS, BSc, PhD, FDS (OS), RCS

*Lecturer in Oral and Maxillofacial Surgery*
*Newcastle University*

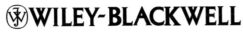

A John Wiley & Sons, Ltd., Publication

This edition first published 2012
© 2012 by Blackwell Publishing Ltd

Wiley-Blackwell is an imprint of John Wiley & Sons, formed by the merger of Wiley's global Scientific, Technical and Medical business with Blackwell Publishing.

*Registered office:*   John Wiley & Sons, Ltd, The Atrium, Southern Gate, Chichester, West Sussex, PO19 8SQ, UK

*Editorial offices:*   9600 Garsington Road, Oxford, OX4 2DQ, UK
The Atrium, Southern Gate, Chichester, West Sussex, PO19 8SQ, UK
2121 State Avenue, Ames, Iowa 50014-8300, USA

For details of our global editorial offices, for customer services and for information about how to apply for permission to reuse the copyright material in this book please see our website at www.wiley.com/wiley-blackwell.

*Library of Congress Cataloging-in-Publication Data*

Dental emergencies / edited by Mark Greenwood.
       p. ; cm.
   Includes bibliographical references and index.
   ISBN 978-0-470-67396-6 (pbk. : alk. paper)
   I. Greenwood, M. (Mark)
   [DNLM: 1. Dental Care-methods.   2. Emergencies.   3. Emergency
Treatment-methods.   WU   105]
   617.6'026-dc23

                                                           2011042659

A catalogue record for this book is available from the British Library.

Wiley also publishes its books in a variety of electronic formats. Some content that appears in print may not be available in electronic books.

Set in 9/12.5 pt Interstate Light by Aptara® Inc., New Delhi, India

1   2012

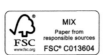

# Contents

# List of Contributors

*U. Chaudhry, BDS, MFDSRCS, DHyp*
Specialist Registrar in Paediatric Dentistry, Manchester Dental Hospital and Royal Manchester Children's Hospital, Manchester

*I.P. Corbett, BDS, BSc, PhD, FDS (OS), RCS*
Lecturer in Oral and Maxillofacial Surgery, Newcastle University, Newcastle

*J. Durham, BDS, PhD, FDS (OS), RCS, FHEA*
Walport Lecturer in Oral and Maxillofacial Surgery, Newcastle University, Newcastle

*J. Greenley, BDS, MFDSRCS*
Senior Dental Officer, Newcastle Dental Hospital, Newcastle

*M. Greenwood, MDS, PhD, FDS, FRCS, FRCS (OMFS), FHEA*
Consultant and Honorary Clinical Professor, Newcastle University, Newcastle

*C.B. Hayward, BDS, Dip Cons Sed*
Associate Specialist, Dental Emergency Clinic, Newcastle Dental Hospital, Newcastle

*I.C. Mackie, BDS, MSc, PhD, FDSRCPS*
Professor and Consultant in Paediatric Dentistry, Manchester Dental School, Manchester

*R.I. Macleod, BDS, PhD, FDSRCS, DDR, RCR*
Consultant in Dental and Maxillofacial Radiology, Newcastle Dental Hospital, Newcastle

*U. J. Moore, PhD, FDSRCS*
Senior Lecturer in Oral Surgery, School of Dental Sciences, Newcastle University, Newcastle

*A. Moufti, DDS, Dip OMFS, PhD, MFDSRCS*
Lecturer in Restorative Dentistry, University of Damascus, Syria

*T. Nugent, BDS, MFDSRCS*
Senior Dental Officer, Community Dental Service, Newcastle

*P.J. Thomson, BDS, MSc, PhD, FFD, FDS, FRCS*
Professor in Oral and Maxillofacial Surgery, Newcastle University, Newcastle

# Preface

The dental emergency clinic is an important area for any dental service. Such departments are usually staffed by clinicians with a variety of backgrounds and levels of experience. This book does not attempt to be exhaustive but is a guide to help clinicians with the management of the wide variety of patients that may present. An attempt is made, where appropriate, to place patient management in an academic context.

# Acknowledgements

Thanks are due to the clinicians and nurses who work on the dental emergency clinic at Newcastle Dental Hospital. We would also like to acknowledge the help given by Mrs Beryl Leggatt in the typing of the manuscript.

Where figures or photographs have been taken from other sources, due acknowledgement is given. Thanks are also due to Dr Anna Beattie and Dr Helen Stancliffe for some of the photographs seen in Chapter 11.

# Chapter 1

# Introduction, Infection Control and Prescribing

## M. Greenwood

## Introduction to the dental emergency clinic

The dental emergency clinic (DEC) is an important part of the service provided to patients. It is a demanding environment in which to work for main two reasons. First, many patients who attend such departments have a general tendency to avoid dental treatment and view attending such a department as a last resort. Second, from the point of view of the clinicians who work in such clinics, the clinical spectrum is wide, and although there is no remit to provide a specialist service, the boundaries of knowledge and experience for clinicians in certain areas are approaching this. Clinical staff working in these departments need a wide skill mix.

This textbook aims to summarise important areas of knowledge with which practitioners working in the DEC should be familiar. Modern clinical working often requires adherence to protocols, and a summary of some of the more important current management protocols, together with supporting evidence, is provided in the appendices.

For maximum efficiency in any department that deals with emergencies, a system of triage is immensely valuable. Triage is essentially the process of determining the priority of patients' treatment on the basis of severity of their condition. Triage should result in determining the order and priority of a patient's emergency treatment and occasionally their onward transport. In the DEC, emergency situations include those where the airway may be compromised due to infection or trauma. Such patients must be assessed promptly and referred quickly for onward management. Other patients, who may have sustained trauma, need to be assessed expeditiously, particularly from the point of view of airway and vital signs, and also possible head injury and concomitant injuries, which in some cases may take priority over the facial

*Dental Emergencies*, First Edition. Edited by Mark Greenwood and Ian Corbett.
© 2012 Blackwell Publishing Ltd. Published 2012 by Blackwell Publishing Ltd.

or dental injuries. More detail in relation to the assessment of trauma patients is given in Chapter 7.

Clearly, it is important that the wide variety and, sometimes, the large number of patients that pass through these departments are handled in an appropriate and a safe manner. In no area does this apply more than the area of infection control, the principles of which are discussed in the following sections.

## Infection and infection control

### Hand care

The most simple and effective method of preventing healthcare-acquired infections is to undertake effective hand hygiene. The World Health Organisation has produced guidelines that have been widely adapted into the '5 moments for hand hygiene'. These are summarised in Box 1.1.

---

**Box 1.1    The 5 moments for hand hygiene at the point of care**

- Before patient contact
- Before aseptic task
- After body fluid exposure risk
- After patient contact
- After contact with patient surroundings

*Source*: Adapted from WHO Alliance for Patient Safety (2006).

---

Handwashing is clearly important in the prevention of spread of infection in general and has received significant media attention in recent years. This is largely due to the prevalence of methicillin-resistant *Staphylococcus aureus* (MRSA). *S. aureus* is a bacterium that lives on the skin and in the nose of approximately one in three of the population. Usually, people who carry MRSA do not require treatment and it is no more likely to cause infection than 'ordinary' *S. aureus*, but different antibiotics are used to treat these patients. Screening for MRSA is carried out for new appointees to healthcare posts and hospital inpatients – but not for outpatients. Effective handwashing is critical in the prevention of spread of MRSA.

The other bacterium that has received significant attention, particularly in recent years, is *Clostridium difficile*. This is a bacterium living in the bowel of less than 5% of the healthy adult population. Patients can develop problems if they are brought into contact with contaminated surfaces (which include hands). Unlike MRSA, alcohol gels are not effective against *C. difficile* spores, and therefore, effective handwashing is mandatory.

It is important that healthcare workers remove all hand jewellery (with the exception of wedding bands), are bare below the elbows and do not wear a wristwatch. All cuts and abrasions should be covered with a waterproof adhesive dressing. It is important that, after handwashing, gloves are worn, and these should be changed between each patient and the hands washed again after removing the gloves. Non-sterile medical gloves can be used for examination purposes, but sterile gloves should be worn for operative procedures.

There is significant individual variation in requirements, but the regular use of an emollient hand cream is important to prevent drying of the skin after frequent handwashing. Contact dermatitis can be significant enough in some practitioners to cause real practical problems with clinical practice. Most organisations now routinely use latex-free gloves as standard.

## Sterilisation and disinfection

**Sterilisation** is defined as the killing or removal of all viable organisms. Concern about the transmissible spongiform encephalopathies such as Creutzfeldt-Jakob disease (CJD) and particularly variant-CJD has improved the level of understanding of prion disease. This has led to a necessary redefinition of sterilisation as the inactivation or removal of all self-propagating biological entities.

**Disinfection** is the reduction in viable organisms to the point where risk of infection is acceptable.

**Antisepsis** is a related term, defined as the disinfection of skin or wounds. It is not practically possible or even necessary to sterilise absolutely everything in a dental surgery. Clearly, all surgical instruments must be sterile and anything coming into direct contact with the surgical site should also be sterile. Everything else should be disinfected.

### Sterilisation and disinfection methods

Before any attempt is made to sterilise or disinfect an instrument, macroscopically evident contamination should be removed. If this is not done, physical access of the sterilising or disinfecting agent to the object being sterilised may be prevented. Therefore, instruments should be pre-cleaned and, if they have been in contact with infectious material, pre-cleaning should include adequate disinfection as a first step.

Methods of sterilisation and disinfection include dry or moist heat, a wide variety of gaseous or liquid chemicals, filtration and ionising radiation. The choice depends largely on the nature of the material being treated, the degree of inactivation required and the organisms involved.

In contemporary practice, procedures are followed that are known to result in sterility for different batch sizes and materials. The performance of equipment in terms of the temperature and duration is carefully monitored. The Bowie-Dick tape is one method of ensuring that an autoclave has been functioning effectively. The cross-hatchings turn brown when sterilisation has

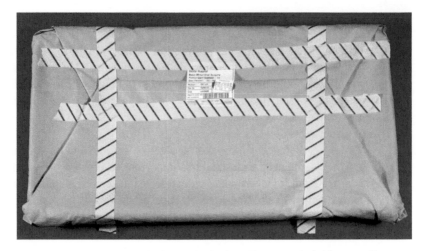

**Figure 1.1** A surgical pack after autoclaving. The cross-hatchings on the Bowie–Dick tape have turned brown indicating that the pack has been successfully sterilised.

been achieved (Figure 1.1). Figure 1.2 shows that the sterilisation has been effective within the packaging itself as the coloured area has changed from yellow to blue.

### Autoclaves

The most common method of sterilisation used in dentistry is by moist heat in an autoclave. The method depends on the use of steam under pressure at temperatures between 121°C and 134°C. It is critical that the autoclave is fully saturated with water vapour and that all other gases are excluded. This method of sterilisation is more efficient than dry heat as it takes less heat to denature fully hydrated proteins and moist heat releases latent heat of vapourisation, which transfers more energy than dry heat.

In some cases, particularly in individuals at high risk from, or those who have known, prion disease, single-use (disposable) equipment should be used wherever possible. Such items include local anaesthetic syringes (Figure 1.3), scalpels, saliva ejectors and impression trays. There is an ever-increasing array of disposable equipment being manufactured.

It is important when dealing with the cleaning of handpieces that the manufacturer's instructions are followed closely. Such equipment should never be completely immersed in disinfectant. It is important to lubricate handpieces appropriately.

Impressions should be rinsed under running cold water to remove macroscopic debris. It is important that further disinfection is carried out according to manufacturer's instructions. The request form to the laboratory that accompanies the impression should highlight known infections or high-risk groups. The same is true of blood samples that are sent for analysis.

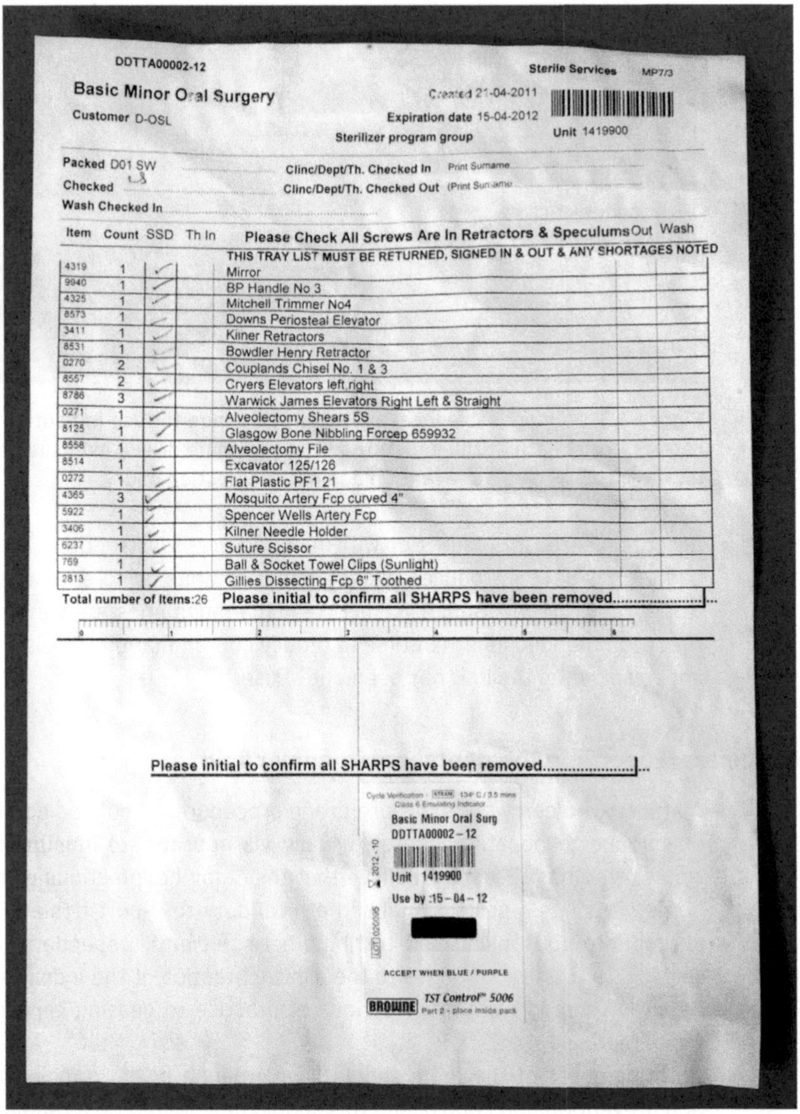

DDTTA00002-12 Sterile Services MP7/3

Basic Minor Oral Surgery

Created 21-04-2011

Customer D-OSL

Expiration date 15-04-2012

Sterilizer program group

Unit 1419900

Packed D01 SW

Checked

Wash Checked In

Clinc/Dept/Th. Checked In Print Surname

Clinc/Dept/Th. Checked Out (Print Surname

Please Check All Screws Are In Retractors & Speculums

THIS TRAY LIST MUST BE RETURNED, SIGNED IN & OUT & ANY SHORTAGES NOTED

| Item | Count | SSD | Th In | | Out | Wash |
|---|---|---|---|---|---|---|
| 4319 | 1 | ✓ | | Mirror | | |
| 9940 | 1 | ✓ | | BP Handle No 3 | | |
| 4325 | 1 | ✓ | | Mitchell Trimmer No4 | | |
| 8573 | 1 | ✓ | | Downs Periosteal Elevator | | |
| 3411 | 1 | ✓ | | Kilner Retractors | | |
| 8531 | 1 | ✓ | | Bowdler Henry Retractor | | |
| 0270 | 2 | ✓ | | Couplands Chisel No. 1 & 3 | | |
| 8557 | 2 | ✓ | | Cryers Elevators left,right | | |
| 8786 | 3 | ✓ | | Warwick James Elevators Right Left & Straight | | |
| 0271 | 1 | ✓ | | Alveolectomy Shears 5S | | |
| 8125 | 1 | ✓ | | Glasgow Bone Nibbling Forcep 659932 | | |
| 8558 | 1 | ✓ | | Alveolectomy File | | |
| 8514 | 1 | ✓ | | Excavator 125/126 | | |
| 0272 | 1 | ✓ | | Flat Plastic PF1 21 | | |
| 4365 | 3 | ✓ | | Mosquito Artery Fcp curved 4" | | |
| 5922 | 1 | ✓ | | Spencer Wells Artery Fcp | | |
| 3406 | 1 | ✓ | | Kilner Needle Holder | | |
| 6237 | 1 | ✓ | | Suture Scissor | | |
| 769 | 1 | ✓ | | Ball & Socket Towel Clips (Sunlight) | | |
| 2813 | 1 | ✓ | | Gillies Dissecting Fcp 6" Toothed | | |

Total number of Items:26 Please initial to confirm all SHARPS have been removed.....................

Please initial to confirm all SHARPS have been removed.....................

Basic Minor Oral Surg

DDTTA00002-12

Unit 1419900

Use by :15-04-12

ACCEPT WHEN BLUE / PURPLE

BROWNE TST Control™ 5006

**Figure 1.2** The sticker at the bottom of the paper has changed from yellow to blue, indicating that sterilisation has been effective within the pack (which is where this form should be placed prior to sterilisation).

## Contamination of surgery water supplies

Most water supplies to dental units will be lined with a biofilm, which provides a reservoir of microbial contamination. Amongst the contaminants is the bacterium *Legionella*, responsible for Legionnaire's disease. Some dental units have a bottle-fed water system, in which case disinfectants can be relatively easily supplied. It is important that manufacturer's instructions are followed. Some of the dental units that are supplied with water more remotely must be

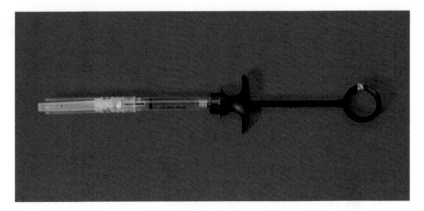

**Figure 1.3** A disposable local anaesthetic syringe for use in dentistry. The retractable sheath at the end of the syringe can be drawn over the needle and locked into place as a prevention against needlestick injury.

decontaminated in conjunction with manufacturer's instructions, and some organisations have introduced decontamination units using ethene oxide plant to perform this function. It is important that such lines are run through for the recommended length of time to reduce contamination. This is particularly important when the unit has been out of use.

## Healthcare workers in the dental emergency clinic

All those who carry out exposure-prone procedures should be non-infectious or immune to hepatitis B virus, usually via appropriate immunisation. Any worker who has reason to believe that they may be infectious with a blood-borne virus has a professional and ethical duty to report this and to obtain appropriate counselling and testing where relevant. Dependent on the result to such testing, changes to the clinical practice of the individual may be required ranging from modifications of practice to ceasing clinical practice altogether.

All members of the team should have training in the principles of infection prevention and control and this should be updated on a regular (usually, annual) basis. It is important that regular reviews are made of the infection control policies and procedures and that these are updated as required.

## Inoculation injuries

Inoculation injuries are defined as incidents where infected objects or substances breach the integrity of the mucous membranes or skin or where a contaminant comes into contact with the eyes.

There are local protocols in place for dealing with such incidents. Clearly, prevention is best and attention to zoning in the surgery ('clean' and 'dirty' areas), and proper disposal of contaminated equipment is vital in this respect.

If such an injury does occur, it is important that the wound is allowed or encouraged to bleed and washed thoroughly with running water. The local protocol should then be followed. Usually, such protocols involve taking blood samples from both the donor (usually, but not always, the patient) and the recipient of the injury (usually, but not always, the clinician). The blood samples should then be tested for blood-borne viruses and, depending on the result, appropriate counselling obtained. The occupational health service should be informed at the earliest opportunity.

## Waste disposal

The safe disposal of waste is critically important in a clinical environment. The main subdivision is into clinical and non-clinical categories. Local protocols may vary but in general terms, clinical waste is disposed of in different coloured plastic bags depending on its nature. It is important that clinicians are familiar with local policies and procedures.

All sharps should be disposed of in a suitable container designed for the purpose. It is important when filling either waste bags or sharps containers that they are not over-filled as this significantly increases the risk of contamination or needlestick injury. Therefore, clinical waste bags must not be filled to a level more than three-quarters full and they should be tied at the neck.

## Blood spillages

Prompt attention is required in the event of a blood spillage. Disposable towels should be placed over the spillage and 10,000 parts per million sodium hypochlorite applied and left for 5 minutes before disposing of the towels as clinical waste. The area should be adequately ventilated, particularly during the cleaning up process. The person clearing such waste should wear appropriate personal protective equipment. In this context, such equipment includes a plastic apron, protective eyewear and heavy-duty gloves. It is advisable to use appropriate protective footwear. Other examples of protective personal equipment are given in Box 1.2.

---

**Box 1.2   Examples of personal protective equipment**

- Gloves
- Protective eyewear (spectacles/visor)
- Masks
- For surgical procedures, clothing protection such as a surgical gown
- Appropriate footwear

## Prescribing

The British National Formulary (BNF) contains excellent guidance on the principles of prescribing. Clinicians in a DEC will need to write prescriptions for some patients and it is important that basic principles are adhered to. An example of a prescription is given in Figure 1.4.

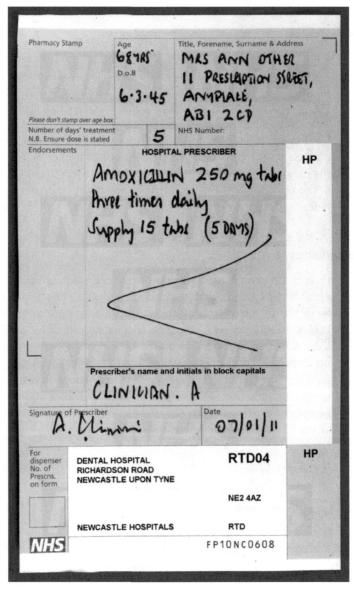

**Figure 1.4** An example of a handwritten prescription. Clearly, such prescriptions should be legible and may be typed, but must be indelible.

Box 1.3 summarises some of the important principles of prescription writing.

---

**Box 1.3   Some basic principles of prescription writing**

- Prescriptions should be written or typed legibly and in indelible ink.
- All areas of the prescription should be completed and signed.
- It is a legal requirement to state the age of children less than 12 years in precise terms.
- The unnecessary use of decimal points should be avoided, e.g. 3 mg not 3.0 mg.
- Use of a decimal point is acceptable to express a range, e.g. 0.5–1 g.
- It is important that figures are placed either side of a decimal point, even if one of the figures is zero.
- Micrograms and milligrams should not be abbreviated as they can easily be misread.
- The dose and frequency should be stated.
- If medications are 'as required', a minimum dose interval must be specified.
- Names of drugs should not be abbreviated.
- Directions should be written in English but the use of well-recognised Latin terms is acceptable, e.g. tds (three times per day), bd (twice per day), qds (four times per day), prn (when required).
- Unlicensed medications (those without marketing authorisation) can be prescribed but the patient should be informed of this.

---

## Antibiotic prescribing

Good infection control and prudent antibiotic prescribing are important in reducing the spread of antibiotic resistance. In many cases of acute oral infections, antibiotics will be required but dental surgeons should not forget important local measures such as irrigation with chlorhexidine where appropriate, together with the removal where possible of the source of infection and provision of drainage where this is possible. Where it is likely that antibiotics are required for a protracted period, or the infection is clinically significant, it is good practice to take a pus swab to send for culture and sensitivity testing. Clearly, if this is done, it is important that the result is checked to ensure that the patient has been prescribed an appropriate antimicrobial (results of culture may take 2–3 days).

In patients who have had previous recent antibiotics or who have a complex medical history that impinges on their overall management, it is important that the clinician working in a DEC discusses the case with a microbiologist, who will provide good advice regarding the best way of managing the patient, particularly from a prescribing viewpoint.

## Prescribing for children

Drug dosages in children are usually based on body weight (measured in kilograms). For many preparations used in dentistry, an age range is used. It is vitally important that the drug dosages are carefully worked out to ensure that they are appropriate. In the BNF, unless the age is specified, the term 'child' applies to persons aged 12 years or less. Dosages according to the age range may vary but the broad age categories are as follows:

- First month (neonate)
- Up to 1 year (infant)
- 1–5 years
- 6–12 years

## Prescribing in the elderly

Older people are often taking multiple medications, which increases the likelihood of drug interactions. Altered pharmacokinetics often result in increased sensitivity of older people to the action of drugs. Even in the absence of known renal disease, renal function deteriorates with age, resulting in reduced drug excretion. Hepatic function also declines with similar potential effects. Low concentrations of serum albumin in chronic ill health can lead to increased free concentrations of protein-bound drugs. Drug absorption is often relatively normal, and therefore, older people often need lower doses, particularly of those drugs that have a narrow therapeutic window.

In the Dental Practitioners Formulary, most antibiotics can be prescribed for the elderly at standard doses. Older patients may be taking iron or calcium preparations, which can impair absorption of tetracyclines. Non-steroidal anti-inflammatory drugs (NSAIDs) should be used with caution, especially in patients who report dyspepsia, have renal disease or cardiac disease requiring treatment with angiotensin-converting enzyme inhibitors. Older people are particularly prone to side effects from drugs that act on the central nervous system, leading to potential confusion, drowsiness and falls.

Elderly patients with impaired vision, mental function or manual dexterity may lead to problems with compliance. It is important that this is borne in mind when prescribing for elderly patients. A summary of points to bear in mind when prescribing for the elderly is given in Box 1.4.

## Prescribing in pregnancy

All drugs should be considered to be potentially teratogenic and should, therefore, be avoided wherever possible. This is particularly the case in the first trimester. The BNF should be checked before any prescription is written for a pregnant patient.

The use of adrenaline-containing local anaesthetics is acceptable in pregnant patients. The optimum time for treatment is the second trimester as the

> **Box 1.4   Considerations in prescribing for the elderly patient**
>
> - Ensure that the patient's current treatment regimen and medical conditions are known.
> - A tendency to use lower doses, particularly of drugs that affect the CNS.
> - Bear in mind potential difficulties with compliance (child-proof drug bottles with tops that an elderly person cannot remove).
> - The British National Formulary has an informative section on prescribing for the elderly, which should be consulted in cases of doubt.

danger is least to the foetus at this time. A hypersensitive gag reflex may be observed in some pregnant patients, which may lead to practical difficulties in treatment.

Intravenous sedation must be avoided in the first trimester and the last month of the third trimester and ideally should be avoided altogether in a pregnant patient. Although nitrous oxide does not appear to be teratogenic, it can interfere with vitamin $B_{12}$ and folate metabolism and should not be used in the first trimester. If it is used at all, the duration of use should be less than 30 minutes, repeated exposure should be avoided and at least 50% oxygen should be administered.

### Breast-feeding
Some drugs can be transferred to the baby in breast milk. The BNF contains a section stating which drugs are implicated.

## Prescribing in hepatic impairment

Liver disease is an important consideration when prescribing drugs. There are a variety of potential reasons for this as summarised in Box 1.5.

> **Box 1.5   Considerations in prescribing for patients with hepatic impairment**
>
> - Impaired drug metabolism.
> - *Hypoproteinaemia*: Reduced protein binding of some drugs leading to increased toxicity.

- *Fluid overload*: Oedema arising from chronic liver disease can be exacerbated by drugs with a tendency to lead to fluid retention, e.g. NSAIDs.
- *Hepatic encephalopathy*: Impairment of cerebral function, e.g. sedatives, opioids.
- *Impaired clotting*: Increases sensitivity to oral anticoagulants.
- Drugs that are hepatotoxic.

## Prescribing in renal impairment

In renal disorders, special consideration needs to be given when prescribing drugs. Clearly those that are excreted by the kidney are important here, but some drugs may be nephrotoxic themselves. The main points are summarised in Box 1.6.

**Box 1.6   Considerations in prescribing for patients with renal disease**

- Side effects of drugs are often tolerated poorly by patients with renal impairment.
- Reduced renal excretion may increase toxicity or the drug itself may be potentially nephrotoxic.
- Sensitivity to some drugs is increased and some drugs become ineffective.

## Conclusions

It is important that all healthcare workers in the DEC are informed about safe practice in the infection control context. Adherence to good practice minimises risk to patients and staff alike.

When prescribing for patients, it is important that basic principles are borne in mind. In any case of doubt, the BNF or equivalent publication must be consulted.

## Further reading

British National Formulary. http://bnf.org.

# Chapter 2

# History Taking and Clinical Examination of Patients on a Dental Emergency Clinic

## I.P. Corbett, C.B. Hayward and M. Greenwood

## Introduction

This chapter outlines a system of history taking and examination of patients attending the dental emergency clinic (DEC) and issues related to consent.

## History taking

This should include the following:

- Demographic data
- Presenting complaint (the presenting problem, ideally recorded in the patient's own words)
- History of presenting complaint (a detailed history of the complaint and the symptoms associated with it recorded in a logical and chronological manner)
- Dental history
- Medical history (current and past)
- Social and family history

### Obtaining information

The initial step in any patient contact is to confirm their identity. It is not unknown in a busy clinic to have two patients with the same surname, or indeed the same forename and surname. In addition, the clinician should introduce themselves and give their designation or grade, in order that the patient knows

*Dental Emergencies*, First Edition. Edited by Mark Greenwood and Ian Corbett.
© 2012 Blackwell Publishing Ltd. Published 2012 by Blackwell Publishing Ltd.

to whom they are talking. It is also good practice to introduce other people who may be present, which may help to lessen the patient's anxiety.

It is important to establish that the advice being sought is for the patient and not for another person, friend or family member. It is also important to ensure that the person with the presenting problem is allowed to speak for themselves. In a multi-cultural society, this may require the use of interpreting services. Such services can be provided by an independent interpreter, a family member in the surgery, or by telephone, for example using 'language lines'. There are possible problems with using a family member for this purpose; the interpretation may be inaccurate, or the family member may not interpret faithfully, in order to manipulate the treatment for reasons that may not be in the patient's best interests. Where an interpreter has been used, this should be carefully documented.

## Demographic data

Demographic data are necessary to identify the correct patient and corresponding clinical record. The minimum data required include the following:

- Title (Mr, Mrs, Ms, Miss, etc.)
- Name (both forename and surname)
- Marital status
- Date of birth
- Sex
- Occupation
- Current address and contact telephone numbers
- Name and contact details of the patient's general medical/dental practitioner (GMP/GDP)

Many organisations may require further data such as ethnicity, religion, NHS number or insurance details. Most DECs will also generate a unique patient identification number in order to reference or cross-reference the patient's attendances.

Data obtained must be recorded accurately and consistently to avoid the inadvertent duplication of records: an example might be 'Mc' used instead of 'Mac' in the case of McDonald or Macdonald.

Some conditions are correlated with age, sex, ethnicity or occupation, and demographic data may help to diagnose a presenting condition more easily, for example a heavy metal worker with dark blue staining at the gingival margins.

## Factors to consider in history taking

History taking is a skill that requires practice. Patients respond in different ways to similar lines of questioning, and it may be necessary to modify questioning style or to ask the same question several times but in different ways in order to optimise the information obtained.

The medical and dental professions are often poor listeners and interject at the earliest opportunity. Although practitioners are all familiar with patients who present their 'life story' following the practitioner's opening question, much important information may be lost by frequent interruptions or curtailing the patient's answers. Other reasons for poor history giving by the patient may include fear or apprehension about treatment, anxiety around hospital-type situations, the so-called 'white coat syndrome'. A perceived lack of confidentiality or an unwillingness to disclose information in front of a parent or other family member may prevent a patient from talking freely. Some patients may have a fear or embarrassment about their condition or what the clinician might say. The patient may misguidedly think that the requested information does not matter or is no business of the clinician. In such cases, the practitioner needs to be persistent in obtaining the information and reassure and explain to the patient why the information is being requested. The clinician may need to take the case history in a more private situation with only a member of staff present to chaperone.

## Components of the history

### Presenting complaint and history of presenting complaint

Patients attending a DEC often present complaining of pain. In order to reach a reliable differential diagnosis or diagnosis, it is important to obtain as far as possible a clear description of the pain. Where possible, use open questions and avoid prompting the patient; for example, 'What does the pain feel like?' is preferable to 'Is the pain sharp or dull?', which restricts and influences the patient response. Once a description of the pain has been obtained, more specific questions can then be used to develop the history further. Basic questions that should be asked are summarised in Box 2.1.

---

**Box 2.1  Points in the history of a patient in pain**

- Site of pain (ask the patient to point with one finger to the place of maximum pain).
- Ask the patient if the pain radiates anywhere.
- Get the patient to describe the pain, e.g. dull ache, sharp, throbbing or shooting.
- Is the pain intermittent or constant? How frequent is it?
- Onset – gradual or sudden?
- Is there anything that makes the pain better or worse?
- What treatments has the patient tried and were they effective?
- Is there a diurnal variation in the pain?
- Does the pain keep the patient awake at night or wake them from sleep?
- Is the pain affected or initiated by hot or cold stimuli?
- Are there any associated symptoms such as swelling, numbness or pain elsewhere?

It is particularly worth asking the patient about the efficacy of analgesics or other treatments that they may have tried as this can sometimes give an indication about the severity of the problem, as highlighted in Box 2.1.

If patients have been subjected to an alleged assault or are injured in any other way, it is particularly important to record comprehensive details of the incident as these may become subject to a legal enquiry at a later stage. Important questions to ask in such situations are summarised in Box 2.2.

---

**Box 2.2   Important questions to ask an injured patient**

- Time and place of alleged assault/injury.
- Was the assailant known to the patient?
- Was there any loss of consciousness?
- Was the patient under the influence of alcohol?
- Were there any other injuries to the body?
- Were there any witnesses? (In particular, if consciousness is in doubt.)
- Were any weapons used?
- What happened immediately after the assault? For example, did the patient attend an accident and emergency department, home or other place, and how did they get there?
- Are the police involved or likely to become involved?
- Note any 'old' injuries, for example a tooth previously fractured or previous facial injuries.

---

### Past and current medical history

The past and current medical history is a description of previous and current medical issues. A systematic approach to data collection is required. The use of a medical history pro forma, often completed by the patient prior to the consultation, may assist in collecting information. However, it is important to go through the collected information carefully with the patient in order to identify any areas of confusion or omission. The medical history should be carefully recorded. Although it is generally only necessary to record positive findings, some practitioners record both negative and positive findings as an aide-memoire to history taking.

Relating the history to the systems of the body is a useful systematic method of questioning the patient on their health and for recording information (see Table 2.1).

It is important to place the patient's medical issues into both medical and social contexts. Many patients and their families live with chronic medical and social conditions and are used to dealing with related problems. The degree of severity of a medical problem can be judged by asking further questions. For example, in patients with epilepsy, the frequency and severity of the

**Table 2.1** Example of a systemic approach to medical history taking.

| System | Examples of problems encountered |
| --- | --- |
| Cardiovascular | Myocardial infarction, angina, hypertension, etc. |
| Respiratory | Asthma, COPD, etc. |
| Gastrointestinal | Peptic ulceration, inflammatory bowel disease, e.g. Crohn's disease, ulcerative colitis |
| Hepatic | Primary and secondary disease, biliary or other cirrhosis, hepatitis |
| Haematological | Blood borne viruses, e.g. hepatitis A/B/C, HIV, clotting disorders, leukaemia, porphyria, sickle cell problems, anaemia |
| Neurological | Epilepsy, cerebrovascular disease, vCJD, psychological/psychiatric disorders |
| Musculoskeletal | Muscular dystrophy, joint replacements, locomotor difficulties |
| Genitourinary and renal | Prostatic disease, genitourinary infection, renal disease or failure, renal transplant, etc. |
| Drug history | Prescribed, non-prescribed, 'recreational' IV drug abuse |
| Allergy | Drugs, Elastoplast®, latex, etc. |
| Past hospitalisation | Medical/surgical |
| Social history | Occupation |
| | Smoking habits; duration, frequency and type |
| | Alcohol consumption: type and quantity |
| | Home and family circumstances |

This table is NOT exhaustive.
COPD, chronic obstructive pulmonary disease; vCJD, variant-Creutzfeldt–Jakob disease.

problem should be ascertained using key questions such as: What medications do you take? What symptoms do you get prior to a seizure? When was your last seizure? Have you been treated in an accident and emergency unit or admitted to a hospital following a seizure? Are you looked after by your GMP or by a specialist? If the clinician has this information, a simple risk assessment can be made, and in the event of a seizure, emergency care is facilitated and a specialist's help more easily obtained if required.

A thorough medical history may uncover conditions that are relevant to diagnosis of the presenting complaint, for example oral ulceration in a patient taking the potassium channel activator nicorandil, or to the subsequent management of the patient, such as alcoholic cirrhosis in a patient requiring extractions. Clearly, patients taking the anticoagulant warfarin require special consideration. This is highlighted in Appendix 3. It is important to remember that warfarin interacts with many of the drugs that dentists can prescribe, and if in doubt, the British National Formulary should be consulted.

Patients who have a high alcohol intake may also have problems with co-agulation. In such cases, if surgical treatment is contemplated, blood should be taken for a full blood count (principally to check the platelet count) and a clotting screen.

# Patient examination

The examination should start from the moment the patient walks into the surgery. Observation of any overt physical or possible psychological disease should be noted. This may manifest in the way a patient moves or walks, their demeanour or relationship with an accompanying family member or person.

The clinician should remember to examine both the normal and affected sides, and record findings, both positive and negative. Examination should be systematic; it is easy to be distracted by an obvious problem and miss a more subtle but possibly more important sign. A full primary examination should be completed before returning to the presenting complaint.

The examination is best divided into an extra-oral examination, followed by intra-oral examination.

## Extra-oral examination

The extra-oral examination starts with a visual examination of the head and neck with particular note made of swellings or deformity, asymmetry of the face, abnormal colour or scars on the skin or lips. In cases of trauma or assault, all soft tissue lacerations, bruising and other related findings must be recorded in detail. A clinical photograph is a useful way of recording information; a diagram can also be made on either a pro forma or freehand sketch, paying particular attention to the abnormal area(s).

Where appropriate, a gross examination of the cranial nerves should be performed, particularly in cases of trauma and infection or if there are other manifest indications, for example in the case of a suspected malignancy.

### Examination of cranial nerves

A detailed system of examination of all the 12 cranial nerves is beyond the scope of this text. A summary of potential cranial nerve problems and basic testing is given in Table 2.2.

After recording the clinical findings, the operator might be in a position to make a definitive diagnosis, a provisional diagnosis or a differential diagnosis. If further investigations are required, the patient may undergo radiography (see Chapter 3) or other special tests such as biopsy, blood tests or tooth vitality tests, for example.

**Swellings**, lumps or bumps should be described following a logical system of site, size, shape, surface, edge, fixation, colour and consistency. Is it a lone-standing lesion or one of multiple lesions? Lesions may be soft or hard. They may be as hard to the touch as bone, or soft (like relaxed muscle) or very soft (like fat). Is the lump pulsatile or fluctuant? Fluid-filled lesions are

**Table 2.2** Cranial nerve problems and examination.

| Cranial nerve | Possible problem | Sign |
|---|---|---|
| I: olfactory | Cranial trauma or tumour | Inability to smell substances |
| II: optic | Facial trauma, tumour, stroke, multiple sclerosis | Decreasing acuity, blindness, visual field defects |
| III: oculomotor | Diabetes, increased intra-cranial pressure | Dilated pupils, ptosis |
| IV: trochlear | Trauma | Diplopia |
| V: trigeminal | Sensory-idiopathic, trauma IDN/lingual nerve damage motor-bulbar palsy, acoustic neuroma, but also signs in cranial nerves VII, IX, X, XI and XII NB: acoustic neuroma also affects VIII | Sensory deficit on testing |
| VI: abducent | Multiple sclerosis, some strokes | Eye unable to look laterally, deviates to the nose |
| VII: facial | LMN – Bell's palsy, skull fracture, parotid tumor UMN – stroke, tumour | Total facial weakness on the affected side (LMN) Forehead spared (UMN) |
| VIII: vestibulocochlear | Noise damage, tumour, acoustic neuroma, Paget's disease of bone | Deafness |
| IX: glossopharyngeal | Trauma or tumour | Impaired gag reflex |
| X: vagus | Trauma or brain stem lesion | Impaired gag reflex, soft palate moves to good side on saying 'ah' |
| XI: accessory | Polio, stroke | Weakness turning head away from affected side |
| XII: hypoglossal | Trauma or brain stem lesion | Tongue deviates to affected side on protrusion |

IDN, inferior dental nerve; UMN, upper motor neurone; LMN, lower motor neurone.

often described as being fluctuant. Fluctuance is the sensation felt when the lesion is palpated between two fingers and a third finger is pressed centrally on the lesion producing a wave-like sensation. Fluid-filled lesions may often be described as 'tense' when they expand and stretch the overlying tissue. Pulsatile lesions must be checked; is the pulsation from the lesion itself or from a deeper lying artery? Swellings may be warm/hot to the touch when involving blood or infection. Involvement of overlying tissues and fixation to deeper structures should be considered (see Chapter 4). Is there any associated lymphadenopathy?

**Temporomandibular joints (TMJs)** should be examined for tenderness on palpation and pain, clicking or crepitus during movement. The TMJ is found anterior to the external auditory meatus and can be simply located by placing a finger over the joint and asking the patient to open and close their mouth to define the position. The condyle can be felt to move. Clicks or crepitations on movement can be felt through the fingertips, or on occasion heard. The path of mandibular movement on opening and closure of the mouth can be observed from the front and from above the patient. Any deviations, restrictions, crepitations or clicks during opening or closing should be recorded, with particular reference to timing in the cycle of mouth opening and closing or on excursive movements. Limitation of opening may be recorded in terms of finger widths or more accurately using a ruler or bite gauge. The TMJs should be examined with care in patients who have been subjected to trauma as they may be involved. In particular, the joints may be involved in whiplash-type injury.

The term 'whiplash' is used to describe the characteristic movement of the head and neck that occurs when the relatively rigid thorax is suddenly subjected to acceleration or deceleration independently of the head. Essentially, it refers to a hyperextension/hyperflexion injury to the soft tissues of the neck. In whiplash, after the neck has been hyperextended, a recoil injury occurs when the neck hyperflexes. As with all injuries, it is important that accurate and contemporaneous records are kept. The injuries in whiplash may be to the bone, soft tissue or both, and a wide variety of clinical manifestations are seen that can be grouped together as 'whiplash associated disorder'. Symptoms in this disorder vary widely and may not be detectable by imaging or physical examination.

In cases where patients present with clinical signs and symptoms of temporomandibular disorder (TMD) following a whiplash injury, the TMD should be treated as in any other of its manifestations, but where there was no previous history, this possibility of aetiology or exacerbation should be borne in mind. If the trauma has been causative, patients may become aware of acute symptoms immediately following the accident. Such symptoms could include an inability to chew and to open the mouth comfortably. It is not uncommon for the patient to develop a TMJ click after such injury. In view of the fact that trauma patients may have several areas of pain and discomfort, symptoms of TMD might not become apparent until much of the 'competing pains' have abated.

## Examination of muscles of mastication

There are many muscles that help in the process of mastication. The main muscles of mastication are four paired muscles: masseter, temporalis, lateral pterygoid and medial pterygoid.

### Masseter muscle

With the teeth clenched and using a hand either side, the masseter muscle is palpated on both sides; from the origin of masseter along the zygomatic arch to the insertion on the ramus and body of mandible.

Masseter is often tender in the central fibres near its insertion. Masseteric pain is associated with parafunctional habits such as bruxism and clenching. Such activity is commonly associated with pain in temporalis.

### Temporalis

The temporalis muscle is palpated in a similar fashion to masseter with the teeth in contact. The muscles should be palpated and tenderness in temporalis may indicate interferences with lateral movement of the mandible.

### Lateral pterygoid

The lateral pterygoids cannot be palpated intra-orally. Hypertonicity in this muscle can be detected by asking the patient to move the mandible laterally against the resistance of the operator's hand. This may elicit pain or discomfort from the lateral pterygoid on the opposite side. This muscle is often painful if there are interferences on the opposite or non-working side.

Bilateral pain in the lateral pterygoid muscles when the patient clenches and slides anteriorly may indicate bruxism or clenching.

### Medial pterygoid

Medial pterygoid may be palpated on the medial aspect of the body of the mandible with the mouth open. This is best achieved using a single finger, tracing the muscle from its superficial head on the maxillary tuberosity to its insertion on the medial aspect of the mandible. This examination is difficult due to the site of the muscle and the risks of triggering the gag reflex.

Problems with increased tonicity in this muscle are often expressed as a feeling of fullness in the throat and occasionally difficulty in swallowing.

## Masticatory muscle disorders

Myofascial pain dysfunction syndrome is commonly associated with high stress levels, parafunctional habits and possibly a poor occlusion. A detailed discussion is beyond the scope of this text (see Chapter 6).

**Major salivary glands** should be examined for abnormality in size, shape and function. Examination is usually a two-handed (bimanual) procedure requiring one hand to palpate the gland intra-orally and the other extra-orally. The glands should be noted for any abnormal tenderness or texture. Swellings of the major salivary glands may be diffuse, involving the whole gland, or discrete as in a lesion within the gland. Swellings of the salivary glands should be described as detailed in the preceding text.

Restriction and/or reduction of salivary flow and also the nature of the saliva produced should be considered, but this can be rather subjective. The parotid glands produce a serous, watery secretion. The submandibular glands produce a mixed serous and mucous secretion, and the sublingual glands produce a predominantly mucous secretion. Examination of secretion is best facilitated by drying the orifice with gauze prior to palpation of the corresponding gland or duct. Observation of the initial secretion 'milked' from the gland is important to avoid missing any pus/calculus expelled from the duct.

**Table 2.3** Significance of enlarged nodes.

| Type | Definition | Significance |
|---|---|---|
| Lymphadenitis | Inflammation of a node | Occurs from an infection in the tissues that are drained by a particular node pathway, e.g. local *Staphylococcus aureus* or systemic, e.g. herpes simplex, HIV, infectious mononucleosis |
| Lymphadenopathy | Any disease process involving the nodes | May be related to infection or neoplasia as primary or secondary metastatic disease |
| Permanent enlargement | Benign lymphoid hyperplasia | Scarring replaces the node structure |

Secretion of saliva is under the control of the autonomic nervous system. If there is parasympathetic stimulation, salivary flow is increased. Sympathetic stimulation will reduce salivary flow. Other factors that can alter salivary flow rate include medications such as beta-blockers, tricyclic antidepressants and chemotherapy drugs. Radiotherapy fields involving salivary tissue reduce salivary flow. Psychological factors such as fear will stimulate the sympathetic nervous system and may cause a dry mouth. Therefore, changes in salivary flow and the nature of the saliva produced can be a good indicator of health locally in the salivary gland itself or possibly reflect a systemic problem.

Further examination of the major salivary glands may include imaging using ultrasound scanning, sialography, magnetic resonance imaging or computerised tomography (CT) (see Chapter 3). Biopsy of salivary glands is usually by fine needle aspiration.

### Lymph nodes

The lymph nodes of the head and neck should be examined from behind the patient by having the patient sitting upright with the neck slightly flexed. Nodes palpable due to infection are tender, soft, enlarged and freely moving. Such nodes usually return to normal size post-infection but can remain enlarged for a considerable period, even indefinitely, due to scarring. Nodes palpable due to malignant disease may be fixed to surrounding tissues, non-tender, hard and involve multiple sites (Table 2.3).

Examination of lymph nodes should be systematic and sequential, checking the auricular, parotid, facial regions and the triangles of the neck to ensure that no areas are missed. All significant findings should be recorded in the patient's records.

## Intra-oral examination

The intra-oral examination should include the following structures:

- Lips and commissures, mucosa of the lips, labial and buccal vestibules, buccal and lingual mucosa and the papillae of the parotid ducts
- Gingivae of all teeth from all aspects
- Hard and soft palate
- Tongue (dorsal, ventral surfaces and the lateral borders; including the papillae on the dorsal surface)
- Tonsillar areas including the lingual area and posterior pharynx
- Floor of mouth, submandibular duct and sublingual salivary gland
- Teeth (occlusion, restorations, caries, signs of trauma and the presence and fit of dentures)

The intra-oral examination should start at the lips and a note made of their colour and presence of lesions or ulceration. Deviation of the junction of the vermillion with skin may be an indicator of previous trauma. Over-exposure to ultra violet light can cause loss of definition of the vermillion. A white lesion of the vermillion may represent a pre-malignant disorder and requires further investigation.

The commissures should be examined for cracking, erythema, crusting and discomfort, which might be an indication of a bacterial (*Staphylococcal*) or fungal (*Candida*) infection in angular cheilitis. This condition is particularly relevant in older patients, immunosuppressed patients and those with ill-fitting dentures with a reduction in face height and resultant over-closure.

With the teeth in occlusion, the mucosa of the upper and lower lips can be examined in turn by everting the lips. The buccal, lingual palatal, floor of mouth and labial mucosa should be examined for colour, texture and the presence of swelling, white, raw or speckled patches or ulceration. The floor of mouth is examined with the tongue tip touching the roof of the mouth as this will make the structures of the floor of mouth more easily visible. It may be necessary to move the tongue from side to side to demonstrate all aspects of the floor of mouth. Care should be taken to examine the lingual 'pouch' posteriorly.

All surfaces of the tongue must be examined. The dorsum of the tongue can best be seen by asking the patient to protrude it. The tongue can be held by the operator by wrapping the tongue in gauze, thus preventing it from slipping during examination. The lateral and ventral surfaces of the tongue must also be examined. Bilateral comparison is useful to highlight any abnormality.

On the upper lip, near the vermillion border, there are yellow-white spots in the submucosa, pinhead in size, the so-called Fordyce spots. These are ectopic sebaceous glands that are not associated with hairs and constitute normal anatomy. They are found in 60-75% of adults. Fordyce spots are also found in the buccal mucosa and the anterior pillar of the fauces.

When the lower lip is retracted and dried, small beads of mucous can be seen to be secreted from the minor or accessory salivary glands. If the commissures are retracted, two landmarks are seen in the buccal mucosa: firstly, the opening of the parotid duct opposite the second maxillary molar tooth and, secondly, a white line running from the corner of the mouth posteriorly parallel to and above the occlusal surfaces of the lower teeth. This is the occlusal line and can vary in size possibly due to chronic trauma from the teeth.

The gingivae should be examined for attachment, morphology, colour, texture, hyperplasia and bleeding on probing. Any recession should be noted. The standard of oral hygiene must be noted along with the presence of plaque and calculus. Relevant mobile teeth might be noted at this point. The gingival examination is undertaken using a pocket measuring probe or World Health Organisation's 621 probe if a basic periodontal examination score is to be recorded.

Examination of the teeth is undertaken using a probe and appropriate design of dental mirror. The teeth should be dry when examined and there should be adequate lighting. All the surfaces of the teeth and the restorations should be examined for disease or failure. The tooth examination is visual (direct observation, transillumination or perhaps by staining) and tactile (using the probe, taking care not to break down demineralised enamel by careless investigation of an early carious lesion). The presence and type of denture and any teeth involved in the support or retention of the denture should be noted where relevant. At this stage, the operator should also note the presence of bridges, crowns and implants.

The hard and soft palate can be seen either directly or indirectly using a mirror. The hard palate should be examined for height, colour, contour, rugae, tori, incisive papilla and for any lesions or ulceration. The soft palate is examined for colour, size, shape, petechiae, ulcers, trauma, gag reflex and symmetry of movement. The uvula should be similarly examined.

The oropharynx is examined by depressing the tongue with a mirror or tongue depressor and having the patient say 'ah'. This allows the posterior wall of the oropharynx to be seen. The tonsils should also be examined for colour, size, surface, character and the presence of infection or ulceration. At this point, a dynamic examination of the tongue, soft palate and uvula may be undertaken. Abnormal movement or loss of movement must be recorded as this may be an indication of a neurological deficit or disease. The same can be said for loss in taste sensation.

## Special tests

Special tests in hard tissue pathology usually involve radiographs of the area of interest (see Chapter 3).

Other special tests include the following:

- Vitality testing using electric pulp testers
- Thermal stimulus testing of tooth vitality:
  o Hot, using warmed gutta-percha
  o Cold, using ethylchloride on cotton wool pledgets

- Percussion sensitivity
- 'Tooth sleuth[®]' to investigate a potential fractured tooth
- Biopsy of a soft tissue lesion – fine needle aspiration, incisional or excisional
- Blood tests, e.g. full blood count, liver function tests, coagulation studies, urea and electrolytes, viral antibodies, etc. (see Appendix 1)
- Vital sign testing (particularly when infection is suspected/confirmed) – see Appendix 2

It is not possible to be comprehensive in this text with regard to all the special tests that can be ordered. In the normal course of events, the operator should be able to arrive at either a provisional, differential or definitive diagnosis, having completed a systematic examination. A decision must then be made to either provide appropriate emergency treatment or refer the patient to a specialist for further investigation and diagnosis.

## Record keeping

It is essential that accurate, systematic and contemporaneous notes are made. This will make the diagnosis easier to determine, avoid repetition and ensure prompt and appropriate treatment for the patient. Occasionally, it may be necessary to defend a diagnosis or course of action in the event of a complaint or litigation. This may occur long after completion of treatment. Accurate records are essential to support judgements that were made at the time. Records should be transparent and chronological. Where new information becomes evident, no attempt should be made to amend previous records. A new correctly dated entry, referencing past notes/records, can be made where appropriate. Remember, if it has not been written down, then it is likely to be deemed not to have happened.

## Consent

Obtaining consent from a patient is an important exercise in communication. It must be done on a voluntary basis and it is important to remember that it is a continuing process. The patient must have the capacity to understand why and to what they are consenting. The basic principles of capacity are set out in the Mental Capacity Act of 2005 (see later). For most outpatient examinations, the principle of implied consent is widely used, meaning that if a patient voluntarily attends and lies in the dental chair awaiting examination, they are deemed to have consented. Implied consent may also be assumed for dental procedures to be carried out under local anaesthetic. However, it is important that the practitioner is absolutely certain that the patient under-stands the nature of the proposed treatment and any potential consequences, particularly where the treatment is complex or where the outcome is more uncertain.

Once relevant information about the procedure and its possible consequences (both beneficial and potential complications) is given, the patient must be able to understand and retain that information, believe it and be capable of making a balance of risk versus potential benefit.

Most patients will consent to procedures that are necessary, but it is a fundamental principle that patients with capacity may refuse consent even if that is against their best interests as determined by the practitioner. This principle holds true even in life-threatening situations. It is important in such cases that the practitioner completes full and contemporaneous records explaining the discussions that have taken place, including the reasons for recommending treatment and, if possible, the reason for refusal, if this is known. Likewise, a patient is not allowed to coerce a practitioner into providing treatment that the practitioner considers to be inappropriate.

It is important that patients are given sufficient information to be able to make an informed judgment about the risks and benefits of any proposed procedure. The Bolam test is important in this regard. Practitioners would not be considered as negligent if they act in accordance with practice that would be accepted by a responsible body of fellow professionals.

When obtaining consent, it is important to give patients the opportunity to ask questions as there may be aspects of particular concern to some patients compared with others. An obvious example of this might be a professional musician for whom the potential consequences of tongue or lip numbness after mandibular third molar surgery may have particularly serious consequences. Repetition of important information is always worthwhile as studies have shown that even when significant risks, including some that may be irreversible, are described, only a small proportion of patients recall being informed of these facts.

It is often wrongly assumed that written consent somehow 'proves' that informed consent has been obtained. There is no proof from a consent form that the knowledge needed by the patient has been understood or retained. However, it is important that the consent process is recorded in the clinical notes, and the consent form does serve this purpose but may need to be augmented with further documentation such as a description of the discussion that took place. The Department of Health has produced a guide to consent and the reference is given at the end of this chapter.

Where treatment will involve a financial transaction, it is essential that the patient is also given an estimate of cost prior to the onset of treatment.

The Mental Capacity Act (2005), referred to previously, is an important piece of legislation designed to protect the rights of individuals to make their own decisions and provide guidelines to address this. It was introduced into practice in 2007. The act sets out guidance for decision-making in the case of people who lack decision-making capacity and applies to all patients aged 16 years and above in England and Wales. There are five basic principles of decision-making (Box 2.3). Decision-making is task specific and is relevant only to a specific decision at a given point in time and should not be extrapolated to other decisions in different situations.

> **Box 2.3   The five basic principles of decision-making**
>
> - *Autonomy* : People are presumed to have capacity until proven otherwise.
> - *Decision-making capacity*: It must be maximised as far as possible.
> - An individual has the right to make their own decision even if learned opinion would consider that decision to be unwise.
> - *Best interests*: If a person is found to lack capacity, decisions or actions taken on their behalf should only be taken in their best interests.
> - *Least restrictive*: Where an individual is found to lack decision-making capacity, the least restrictive decision or action should be taken.

The person who is proposing treatment and seeking consent should be the same person who assesses capacity. The critical questions to answer are:

(1) Is there an impairment of, or disturbance in the function of, the mind or brain?
(2) If there is such disturbance, does this impair the individual's ability to make a particular decision?

A four-stage test, adapted from common law, must then be applied to examine the decision-making process. A person is unable to make a decision for themselves if they are unable to:

(1) understand the information relevant to the decision;
(2) retain information (for at least long enough to make the decision);
(3) use or weigh information as part of the process of making the decision;
(4) communicate their decision (by talking, using sign language or any other unambiguous means).

It is important that relevant information is provided in a manner appropriate to the needs of the patient. There is also a requirement to attempt to determine whether a Lasting Power of Attorney exists (appointing someone to act on the patient's behalf in relation to health and welfare decisions).

If there is a problem with an individual's capacity to make a particular decision, there are two courses of action: (1) to defer treatment and reassess or (2) to act in the patient's 'best interests'. Best interests can only be determined on an individual basis and must take into account every possible source of information. This may require the involvement of an Independent Mental Capacity Advocate (IMCA). More detailed information is contained within the Mental Capacity Act and its Code of Practice.

If the clinician feels that a patient should be referred for further assessment due to lack of capacity for psychiatric reasons, there are several potential routes to follow. These are summarised in Box 2.4.

---

**Box 2.4 Possible actions in dealing with a patient with a psychiatric disorder**

- *New presentation of a psychiatric illness*: Such patients should be encouraged to speak to their general medical practitioner (GMP) in the first instance – it may be appropriate not to suggest that the problem might be a psychiatric illness.
- *Deterioration of a known psychiatric illness*: Patients should be asked to speak to their GMP or, if appropriate, existing psychiatric care workers.
- *Overt suicidal ideation*: These patients should be advised to speak to their GMP, but the situation may require immediate attendance at the accident and emergency department or urgent referral to the on-call psychiatric services. In cases of immediate concern, it may be necessary to contact the police.
- *Immediate danger*: In the case of a patient presenting an *immediate danger* to others, call the police or hospital security.

---

## Conclusions

A thorough history and examination is essential for all patients. Even in apparently straightforward cases, going through this process will sometimes reveal that the case may be more complicated than initially thought.

When treatment has been decided upon, it is essential that the patient understands what treatment is going to be carried out, and why it is needed.

## Further reading

Department of Health (2001) Reference guide to consent for examination or treatment. London: Department of Health. www.dh.gov.uk/prod_consum_dh/groups/dh_digitalassets/@dh/@en/documents/digitalasset/dh_4019079.pdf

Greenwood M, Seymour RA, Meechan JG (eds) (2009) Clinical examination and history taking. In: *Textbook of Human Disease in Dentistry*, Chapter 1. Wiley-Blackwell, Oxford.

# Chapter 3

# Radiology and the Dental Emergency Clinic

## R.I. Macleod

## Introduction

X-ray examination is an important tool that helps clinicians to diagnose, plan and monitor both treatment and lesion development. In the United Kingdom, dental radiographs account for approximately one-third of all diagnostic radiological examinations, which emphasises their value in virtually all areas of dental work.

X-rays are part of the electromagnetic spectrum with a high energy and ability to cause ionisation and damage to living tissue. Low-dose damage is cumulative and adverse effects can take decades to become manifest but include the potential development of malignancy. As a consequence, X-rays need to be used prudently. Their use is controlled by specific legislation, which in the United Kingdom includes the Ionising Radiations Regulations 1999 (IRR99) and the Ionising Radiations (Medical Exposure) Regulations 2000 (IR (ME) R2000). Details of these regulations will not be given here but are based on three core concepts of radiation protection: justification, optimisation and limitation, which are discussed in the following sections.

## Justification

The prescription of a radiograph must, in every case, be of some positive benefit to the patient and influence their treatment. The clinician should be sure that the information required is not already available on an existing film or obtainable using any other means. In the dental emergency clinic, this can cause significant inconvenience but the basic principle should be remembered.

*Dental Emergencies*, First Edition. Edited by Mark Greenwood and Ian Corbett.
© 2012 Blackwell Publishing Ltd. Published 2012 by Blackwell Publishing Ltd.

## Optimisation

Where the decision has been made to request a radiograph, the dose must be kept 'as low as reasonably practicable'. This can be achieved by using appropriate equipment, good technique and by having a quality control programme in place to ensure films are consistently of diagnostic quality.

## Limitation

Limitation incorporates the concepts of justification and optimisation and also that all X-ray equipment is operating within accepted dose limits. It is important that X-ray equipment is subject to formal acceptance testing, routine quality control, undergoes proper maintenance and has all the standard dose reduction features present.

An essential aspect of justification for any radiographic examination is that such examination should not be undertaken until after a clinical history and examination has been performed. The concept of 'routine' or 'screening' radiographs should be avoided. Guidelines on the appropriate use of radiographs in dental practice, such as those produced by the Faculty of General Dental Practitioners of the Royal College of Surgeons of England should be followed.

It should be remembered that children are more susceptible to the damaging effects of ionising radiation and consequently their use should be even more circumspect.

There are basically four types of dental radiological procedure:

(1) Intra-oral (bitewing, periapical and occlusal) radiography
(2) Panoramic radiography (DPT)
(3) Cephalometric radiography
(4) Cone-beam computed tomography (CBCT)

Figure 3.1 shows a panoramic radiograph and is labelled to show the features. Generally, where detail is required, such as for the assessment of dental caries, periapical pathology, periodontal assessment or root fractures, intra-oral views are the most useful, whereas if the examination requirement extends beyond purely the dento-alveolar region, extra-oral imaging may be more appropriate. However, extra-oral views have a higher radiation dose.

The increasing use of digital sensors in dental radiography does result in a lowering of dose, particularly for intra-oral radiographs, and also gives the facility for computer manipulation of the images as well as enhancing their diagnostic usefulness. Typical effective doses in dental radiography are shown in Box 3.1.

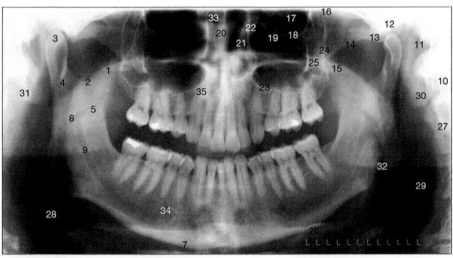

**Figure 3.1** A panoramic radiograph demonstrating the anatomy that can be imaged.

| | | |
|---|---|---|
| 1. Coronoid Process | 13. Articular Eminence | 25. Malar Process |
| 2. Sigmoid Notch | 14. Zygomatic Arch | 26. Hyoid Bone |
| 3. Mandibular Condyle | 15. Pterygoid Plates | 27. Cervical Vertebrae 1–4 |
| 4. Condylar Neck | 16. Pterygomaxillary Fissure | 28. Epiglottis |
| 5. Mandibular Ramus | 17. Orbit | 29. Soft Tissues of Neck (Look Vertically |
| 6. Angle of Mandible | 18. Inferior Orbital Rim | for Carotid Artery Calcification here) |
| 7. Inferior Border of Mandible | 19. Infraorbital Canal | 30. Auricle |
| 8. Lingula | 20. Nasal Septum | 31. Styloid Process |
| 9. Mandibular Canal | 21. Inferior Turbinate | 32. Oropharyngeal Air Space |
| 10. Mastoid Process | 22. Medial Wall of Maxillary Sinus | 33. Nasal Air Space |
| 11. External Auditory Meatus | 23. Inferior Border of Maxillary Sinus | 34. Mental Foramen |
| 12. Glenoid Fossa | 24. Posterolateral Wall of Maxillary Sinus | 35. Hard Palate |

---

### Box 3.1    Effective doses in dental radiography

- Intra-oral dental X-ray imaging procedure 1-8 µSv
- Panoramic examinations 4-30 µSv
- Cephalometric examinations 2-3 µSv
- Cone beam computed tomography procedures 34-652 µSv (for small dento-alveolar volumes) and 30-1079 µSv (for large 'cranio-facial' volumes)
- Natural background radiation 2-8 mSv/year
  (µSv = microsievert)

---

### Cone-beam computed tomography

CBCT offers the dental surgeon a new way to image their patients in axial, coronal and sagittal planes with three-dimensional (3D) reconstructions as well as in variable panoramic slices. The full potential of this technique is still to be fully realised. An example of a CBCT image is shown in Figure 3.2

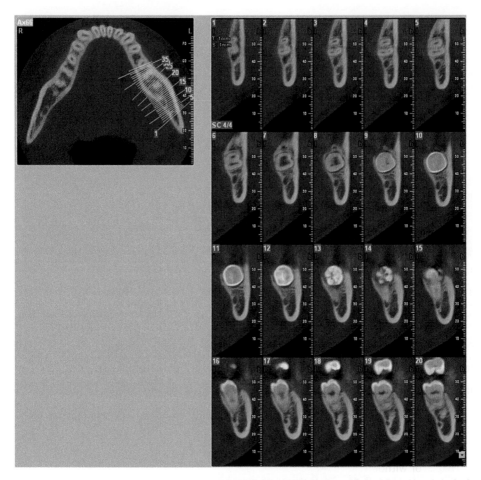

**Figure 3.2** Cone-beam computed tomographic image that shows the detail of anatomy, including its facility for cross-sectional imaging.

demonstrating the detail provided. As equipment becomes more common and affordable, the number of clinical situations when CBCT may be used will increase but it should be remembered that the dose is considerably higher than for other dental imaging modalities. Views such as intra-orals may still be the most appropriate, however in many situations. In general, the following guide for CBCT can be considered.

### Factors to consider in the use of CBCT

The smallest volume compatible with the clinical situation should be used where this provides lower radiation dose to patients. Kilovoltage and milliamperes should be optimised for each clinical application and patient.

Some CBCT systems offer a choice of 'resolution'. The voxel size compatible with the clinical situation should be used where this provides lower radiation dose to the patient.

CBCT systems in many cases allow the operator to opt for imaging based on a reduced number of basis projections. Such options should be used where the resulting image quality is acceptable for the clinical situation.

It should also be considered that with larger volumes, areas of anatomy (and potential pathology) outwith the normal dental remit will be demonstrated and it would be a wise precaution to have such views scrutinised by an appropriately qualified specialist radiologist.

In this chapter, two common areas of emergency clinical presentation, pain and trauma, will be considered.

## Patients in pain

As indicated previously, for dental and peridental tissues, intra-oral views give more detail than extra-oral views and show earlier, more subtle changes, but their use may be limited by the patient's ability to cope with a film in a painful mouth or where there is trismus. In such cases, sectional panoramic views (or small volume CBCT) may provide sufficient evidence of the clinical problem.

### Radiographs useful for the investigation of dento-facial pain

#### Toothache
A periapical view of the tooth under suspicion (Figure 3.3) or bitewing of the affected side.

#### Dental abscess
A periapical view of the affected tooth or sectional panoramic view (DPT) with or without facial swelling.

#### Pericoronitis
A sectional DPT of the affected side should be taken, or full DPT if a problem with both sides and consideration is being given for the removal of all wisdom teeth under general anaesthetic. CBCT can give more information of the position of the tooth and its relation to adjacent anatomical structures such as the inferior dental canal.

#### Sinusitis
Maxillary sinusitis is essentially a clinical diagnosis. Computed tomography (CT) can be useful in more persistent cases following an ENT examination. Occipito-mental views are now considered of little value in this respect. The role of CBCT will probably be similar to CT.

#### Temporomandibular joint imaging
Temporomandibular joint (TMJ) imaging techniques such as a specific DPT programme and CBCT have the ability to demonstrate the TM joint. However, this should only be undertaken if it is likely to influence either the diagnosis

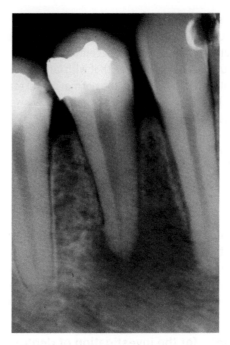

**Figure 3.3** A periapical view of a lower right first premolar showing periapical rarefaction and loss of apical lamina dura. Appearances are consistent with periapical inflammation secondary to a non-vital tooth.

or treatment of the condition. Neither technique demonstrates the articular disc, which is often the source of many of the problems including clicking and locking, as well as pain. The only method that would demonstrate the disc, apart from endoscopy, is magnetic resonance imaging (MRI). In many respects, this can be regarded as the gold standard for TMJ imaging. However, access and cost as well as how such imaging would influence treatment needs to be taken into consideration before referring patients for such investigations.

### Trigeminal neuralgia
Essentially, trigeminal neuralgia is a clinical diagnosis but MRI is indicated to assess for vascular anomalies or neoplasia on or around the trigeminal nerve tract. The presence of multiple sclerosis should be considered in younger patients (<40 years) (see Chapter 6).

### Atypical (Idiopathic facial pain)
Plain films such as a sectional DPT to exclude dental disease should be taken. Possibly MRI to exclude a more central problem, such as neoplasia or cerebrovascular complication should be considered.

### Salivary glands and imaging
Acute sialadenitis requires no imaging. More chronic problems, particularly if intermittent and associated with meals, can be examined using plain films

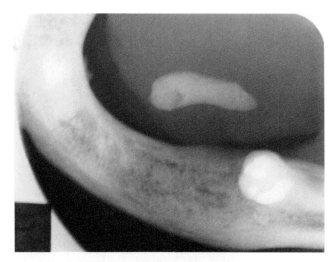

**Figure 3.4** A lower occlusal view showing the presence of a sizeable salivary calculus.

such as a DPT of the affected side plus a lower true occlusal for submandibular calculi (Figure 3.4). Sialography of the affected gland has been the traditional way of investigating the cause of an obstructive sialadenitis but increasingly the use of ultrasound has gained in usefulness as a first-line investigation for many salivary problems. Ultrasound has the advantage that it does not expose the patient to radiation.

## Trauma radiology

All radiographic images are two-dimensional representations of a 3D object. In general, if a fracture is suspected, at least two views at right angles are required in order to determine the presence of a fracture(s), extent and any displacement. In the case of a suspected fractured mandible, a DPT should be obtained, but in addition a postero-anterior view should also be obtained (Figure 3.5). Fractures will not be seen on radiographs where the fracture is oblique to the line of the X-ray beam as the two halves of the fracture will become superimposed and thus become invisible. This problem is commonly seen in root fractures on a periapical film using the paralleling technique as root fractures tend to be diagonal, but where a fracture is clinically suspected, a bisecting angle view (or anterior occlusal view) is more likely to demonstrate it.

When dealing with fractured teeth, the saying 'count and account' should always be remembered (see Chapter 7). Fragments of teeth may end up in the mouth, out of the mouth, swallowed or inhaled! Those in the mouth may be apparent but when traumatically implanted in adjacent soft tissue such as the lip, these areas should be carefully explored and radiographs of the area taken at the lowest exposure setting possible. If there is any suspicion that

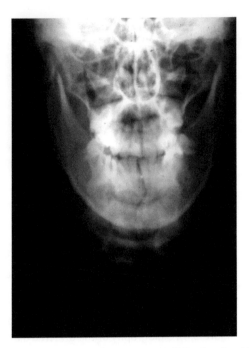

**Figure 3.5** A postero-anterior view of the mandible showing bilateral fractures of the condyles and a midline mandibular fracture. Such a combination of fractures is often referred to as a 'Guardsman's fracture'.

the patient may have inhaled either a complete tooth or tooth fragment they should be sent for appropriate chest radiographs without delay. Swallowed tooth fragments are unlikely to cause any harm unless symptoms supervene and the patient can be reassured with no need for abdominal radiographs. Table 3.1 lists radiographic examinations used in facial trauma cases.

## Looking at radiographs

The clinician is often the only person to evaluate a radiograph, which means it is easy to miss pathology, particularly when unexpected, if the images are sub-optimal in quality or viewed in an inadequate way. Ideal viewing conditions for radiographs should include the following:

- A purpose made light box, preferably with a mask that can exclude surrounding light or using a high-definition monitor for a digital system.
- Magnification, particularly for small dental films, can be useful.
- The room light should be subdued and the operator alert!

Equipment is available commercially to assist practitioners to enable viewing to be conducted in the above manner. If using or considering digital

**Table 3.1** Radiographs useful in the investigation of trauma.

| Type of fracture | Radiographic examination |
| --- | --- |
| Suspected dento-alveolar fracture | See aforementioned notes, but periapicals taken using bisecting angle technique at different angulations or anterior occlusal views plus a periapical. CBCT may be of value in some cases. |
| Suspected mandibular fracture | DPT and postero-anterior mandible views are routine but could be supplemented with a lower true occlusal view if midline fracture is suspected. Reverse Towne's view is a useful view to demonstrate the condyles. CBCT may be of value in assessment of mandibular fractures. |
| Suspected zygomatic fracture | Occipito-mental 10° and 30° supplemented with a modified submentovertex ('jug handle') view if fracture limited to zygomatic arch. CBCT could also be used to assess the zygomatico-maxillary complex. |
| Suspected middle third facial fracture | Facial bone series including occipito-mental 10° and 30° and lateral skull or CT scan. CBCT may substitute conventional CT but would be less beneficial if an intra-cranial complication was suspected. |

CBCT, cone-beam computed tomography; DPT, panoramic radiography; CT, computed tomography.

imaging, careful consideration should be given to the type, size and location of the monitor in the surgery.

Each image should be viewed systematically, ensuring that it is examined in its entirety and avoiding 'tunnel vision' onto just the area of interest. Where there is any uncertainty, check the clinical situation and consider an alternative

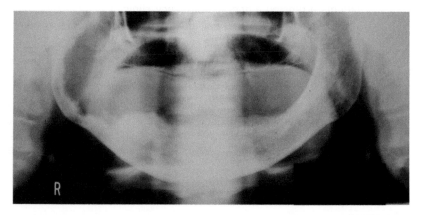

**Figure 3.6** A panoramic radiograph showing gross erosion of the right ramus and body of mandible. This was due to an overlying squamous cell carcinoma.

imaging mode, for example a panoramic view if an area appears to extend beyond the margins of an intra-oral view.

## Interpretation of images

A thorough knowledge of normal radiographic appearances is essential in detecting the abnormal, particularly when looking at more advanced modalities such as DPTs (Figure 3.6) and CBCT views. Features to consider when describing radiographic appearances are summarised in Box 3.2.

---

**Box 3.2   Factors to consider when interpreting radiographic images**

- *Density*: Radio-opaque, radiolucent or mixed
- *Number of lesions*: Whether single or multiple
- *Site*: Anatomical location
- *Size*: Allowing for geometric distortion of the imaging modality used
- *Borders*: Well defined, corticated or ill-defined
- *Internal structure*: Homogeneous, internal calcifications, unilocular or loculated radiolucency
- *Effect on surrounding structures*: Non-apparent, bone expansion, destruction, root resorption or displacement
- *Changes over time*: Look at any previous films available

---

## Conclusions

Radiological investigations are often an essential part of the assessment of patients attending a dental emergency clinic. It is important that clinicians working in such areas are familiar with the principles of these investigations.

## Further reading

Pendlebury ME, Horner K, Eaton KA (eds) (2004) *Selection Criteria for Dental Radiography*. Faculty of General Dental Practitioners (UK) Royal College of Surgeons of England, London.

# Chapter 4

# Acute Oral Medical and Surgical Conditions

## P.J. Thomson

## Introduction

Oral medicine and oral surgery are specialised branches of dentistry that deal with a wide range of disorders affecting the mouth, face and jaws and which normally require medical or surgical intervention. There is considerable overlap in the range of conditions that present to medical and surgical specialists, but a number of very important clinical conditions can present acutely to dental practitioners.

Whilst the detailed management of these disorders is outside the scope of this book, it is important that the dental emergency clinic practitioner is aware not only of the type and medical significance of such presentations, but also which patients should be referred for specialist assessment and treatment. As most dental emergency clinics function as integral parts of dental hospitals, close working relationships exist with oral and maxillofacial surgery units and oral medicine departments that facilitate such care.

An acute condition may be defined as a suddenly presenting disorder, usually with only a short history of symptoms, but with a degree of severity that causes significant disruption to the patient. They include traumatic injuries (described in Chapter 7), facial pain (which is discussed in detail in Chapter 6), swellings arising both intra-orally and around the face, jaws and neck, blistering and ulcerative disorders of the oral mucosa, disturbed oro-facial sensory or motor function and haemorrhage. This chapter will summarise a wide range of clinical disorders that practitioners should be aware of and which may present as acute conditions in the emergency clinic.

## Oro-facial swelling

A swelling is defined as a transient enlargement or protuberance of part of the body and may arise intra-orally or externally around the face, jaws

---

*Dental Emergencies*, First Edition. Edited by Mark Greenwood and Ian Corbett.
© 2012 Blackwell Publishing Ltd. Published 2012 by Blackwell Publishing Ltd.

and neck. Acute swellings are usually caused by trauma, or infection and inflammation.

Traumatic swellings include haematoma, facial or dento-alveolar fractures and temporomandibular joint effusions or dislocations. Signs and symptoms that help the clinician to recognise facial fractures are summarised in Table 4.1. Fractures inevitably display localised swelling, bruising and deformity and the patient will experience both pain and some loss of function. The precise

**Table 4.1**   Signs and symptoms of facial fractures.

| Type of facial fracture | Sign and symptom |
|---|---|
| Unilateral condyle | Fracture side:<br>• Pain, swelling, bruising<br>• Joint immobility<br>• Deviation of mandible on mouth opening<br>• Premature tooth contact<br><br>Opposite side:<br>• Lateral open bite<br>• Inability to move mandible laterally |
| Bilateral condyle | • Pain, swelling, bruising and immobility of both joints<br>• Anterior open bite<br>• No lateral mandibular movement possible |
| Mandible | • Pain, swelling, bruising at site of fracture<br>• Trismus<br>• Abnormal mobility of fractured segments<br>• Step deformity at lower border of mandible<br>• Deranged occlusion<br>• Numbness of lip and chin |
| Zygomatico-orbital complex | • Pain, swelling, bruising over cheek and around eye<br>• Subconjunctival haemorrhage<br>• Later, flattening and depression of cheek prominence<br>• Step deformity at infra-orbital margin<br>• Numbness of upper lip, lateral nose and cheek<br>• Intra-oral bruising in upper buccal sulcus<br>• Trismus if coronoid process impacts on displaced zygoma |
| Middle third fractures | • Can be gross facial swelling and tenderness<br>• Bilateral circumorbital bruising<br>• Mobility at infra-orbital margins or zygomatico-frontal sutures<br>• Widespread facial numbness<br>• Deranged occlusion with anterior open bite<br>• Mobile maxillary alveolus |

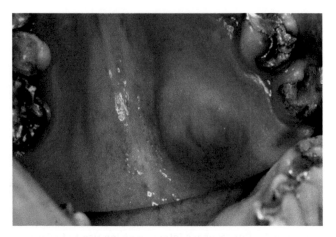

**Figure 4.1** Minor salivary gland tumour arising in palatal tissue.

history of the preceding injury, examination of the anatomical site involved and standard radiographic assessment will help clarify the diagnosis, and these cases should be referred to specialist oral and maxillofacial surgery opinion.

Localised intra-oral swellings are very common, and although sometimes of long standing may present as 'acute' problems due to sudden patient awareness. Gingival swellings may represent localised acute periodontal problems or rarer disorders such as giant cell granulomas, whilst palatal swellings can arise from acute dental abscesses or infected odontogenic cysts, particularly involving the lateral incisor or palatal roots of molar teeth, but may be due to other more sinister causes such as minor salivary gland tumours. Tumours arising from minor salivary glands are often malignant and the practitioner should have a high index of suspicion, especially for diffuse, firm palatal swellings in the absence of obvious dental disease. Figure 4.1 illustrates a salivary gland tumour arising in the palate.

Similarly, patients may present with lip swellings that may be diffuse or more localised. Acute, diffuse lip swelling usually represents an allergic response but localised lesions may arise from inflammation or obstruction of minor salivary gland lesions. Whilst mucus extravasation cysts, due to local trauma, account for the majority of lower lip lesions, upper lip swellings are more commonly the result of minor salivary gland tumours.

Acute inflammatory and infective swellings may arise in a number of anatomical sites around the mouth and face, presenting intra-orally as localised dental abscesses or cervico-facial swellings due to spreading tissue space infections. Figure 4.2 shows facial swelling characteristic of a buccal space infection following an intra-oral dental abscess. The various types of clinical presentation, the anatomical sites where infections can localise and their relevant diagnostic features are summarised in Table 4.2.

The rapid spread of infection through connective tissue spaces, often referred to as cellulitis, can give rise to airway obstruction and life-threatening conditions, such as Ludwig's angina, which is a large infective swelling

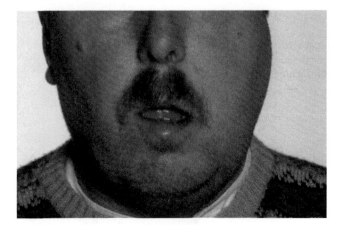

**Figure 4.2**   Buccal space infection giving rise to facial swelling.

involving bilateral submandibular, sublingual and submental spaces. Swelling may extend down the anterior neck, with massive distension of the floor of the mouth and elevation and protrusion of the tongue. *Such presentations are acute surgical emergencies and require immediate referral.*

The cardinal signs of acute inflammation comprise swelling (often with resultant suppuration and abscess formation), pain, redness, heat and loss of function. Sometimes, patients may present with cutaneous swellings or sinuses as a result of discharge of infected material from dental abscesses. There may also be systemic signs such as pyrexia, malaise, sweating, dehydration and rapid pulse.

Clearly, clinical management is dependent upon the precise cause of infection and the general state of the patient. Localised dento-alveolar abscesses may be appropriately treated by intra-oral drainage via tooth extraction, opening of root canals and/or intra-oral incision and drainage. Wherever there are signs of spreading cervico-facial infection or significant systemic disturbance, however, patients should be referred urgently to the maxillofacial unit for admission and further management.

One of the commonest acute oral surgery conditions to present to the emergency clinic is pericoronitis, inflammation around the crown of a partly erupted or impacted tooth usually the mandibular third molar. In acute cases, the patient experiences pain and swelling around the tooth, together with a foul taste and often halitosis. There may also be trismus, dysphagia, facial swelling and pyrexia. Diagnosis follows radiographic examination and confirmation that the infection has not arisen from infected adjacent teeth. Extraction of traumatic upper third molars, localised antibacterial treatment and antibiotic prescription may be required to ease the acute condition before referral for specialist advice on surgical removal. As in all infective conditions, *rapidly spreading facial or neck swelling requires urgent referral and hospital admission.*

A number of acute oral mucosal infections, such as pseudomembranous candidiasis or herpetic gingivostomatitis may give rise not only to classical

**Table 4.2** Oro-facial tissue space infections.

| Anatomical site | Location | Clinical signs |
|---|---|---|
| *Lower jaw tissue spaces* | | |
| Submental | Between mylohyoid above and skin below | Firm swelling beneath chin |
| Submandibular | Between anterior and posterior digastric muscles | Submandibular swelling |
| Sublingual | Lingual mandible between mylohyoid and mucosa | Floor of mouth swelling and raised tongue |
| Buccal | Between buccinator and masseter | Swelling behind angle of mouth to lower mandibular border |
| Submasseteric | Between masseter and lateral ramus | Trismus, swelling confined to masseter |
| Pterygomandibular | Between medial pterygoid and medial ramus | Severe trismus, dysphagia, limited buccal and submandibular swelling |
| Lateral pharyngeal | Skull base to hyoid, medially pharyngeal muscle, laterally fascia | Pyrexia, malaise, dysphagia, trismus, swollen fauces |
| Peritonsillar | Between pharyngeal muscle and tonsil | Dysphagia, 'hot potato' speech, swollen fauces and soft palate |
| *Upper jaw tissue spaces* | | |
| Lip | Between orbicularis oris and mucosa | Diffuse labial swelling |
| Canine fossa | Between levator muscles and facial skin | Diffuse swelling lip, cheek and lower eyelid |
| Palatal | Subperiosteal space | Circumscribed fluctuant palatal swelling |
| Infratemporal fossa | Below greater wing of sphenoid, ramus lateral and pterygoid plate medial | Trismus, pyrexia |
| Subtemporalis | Between temporal bone and temporalis muscle | Temporal swelling, trismus |

intra-oral discomfort or ulceration but also to labial and facial swelling and cervical lymphadenopathy.

Acute swelling of the major salivary glands may also present to the dental emergency clinic. Whilst an acute bacterial parotitis, usually a consequence of dehydration or obstructed salivary flow, is rarely seen these days, viral parotitis due to mumps infection is becoming more common. In the UK, in particular, this may be related to a lack of uptake of the MMR vaccine due to adverse publicity in the late 1990s. Whilst the classic description of mumps

**Table 4.3** Differential diagnosis of neck lumps.

| Type of lump in next | Cause |
| --- | --- |
| Skin and superficial fascial lesions | Infective skin lesions<br>Epidermoid cyst<br>Lipoma |
| Cystic lesions | Sublingual dermoid<br>Thyroglossal cyst<br>Branchial cyst<br>Lymphangioma |
| Cervical lymphadenopathy | Acute lymphadenitis<br>Chronic infections<br>Metastatic malignant disease<br>Leukaemia or lymphoma |
| Others | Thyroid gland disease<br>Aneurysm<br>Sternomastoid tumour<br>Cervical rib<br>Carotid body tumour |

emphasises bilateral parotid swelling with everted earlobes and accompanying submandibular swelling, patients often present initially with an acute unilateral parotid swelling that may pose a diagnostic dilemma.

Isolated acute submandibular salivary gland swellings are less common, more usually presenting as intermittent obstructive swellings due to calculus formation in the ductal system. The history and clinical examination is usually sufficient to establish the diagnosis. Salivary gland disorders are best referred to oral and maxillofacial surgery specialists for further investigation and management.

Swellings may also present as more discrete neck lumps. Whilst there is a wide range of causes for a lump in the neck, summarised in Table 4.3, many of these may be long-standing, chronic disorders that have only just been noticed by the patient. Most patients are well aware of the potential sinister nature of lumps and will usually be anxious. The salient features to ascertain on examination of neck lumps are summarised in Box 4.1.

Acute cervical lymphadenopathy is not a common presentation in dental emergency clinics but can arise as a result of bacterial infection anywhere in the head and neck, viral infections such as infectious mononucleosis, rubella or cat scratch fever, unusual infections such as toxoplasmosis or as a result of haematological malignancies such as acute leukaemia or lymphoma. In the absence of an obvious dental cause, investigation and management of neck lumps is a surgical problem and appropriate referral to a maxillofacial unit is essential.

**Angioedema** is a rare, immune-mediated disorder that gives rise to a rapid, oedematous swelling of the face, particularly involving the lips or tongue. Figure 4.3 demonstrates the acute, transient diffuse swelling of the

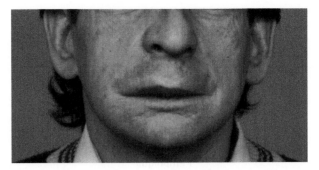

**Figure 4.3** Angioedema producing characteristic acute swelling of the upper lip and face.

---

**Box 4.1   Examination of a neck lump**

- Anatomical site, tissue of origin and depth
- Single or multiple
- Associated cervical lymphadenopathy
- Size (measure accurately)
- Shape
- Surface - smooth/lobulated/irregular
- Edge - defined/diffuse
- Colour
- Consistency - soft/firm/rubbery/hard
- Tender or warm on palpation
- Fluctuation
- Transillumination
- Pulsation
- General condition of the patient - well/pyrexial/cachexic

---

upper lip so characteristic of angioedema. It may be allergic in origin due to a type I hypersensitivity reaction or hereditary as a result of complement C1 esterase inhibitor deficiency. Although often transient and self-limiting, resolving spontaneously over a few hours, oedema may spread to the neck and threaten the airway. Whilst mild cases may be managed in the emergency clinic with reassurance and/or the use of oral antihistamines, more severe cases should be treated as acute anaphylactic reactions and referred to oral and maxillofacial surgery.

## Blistering disorders of the oral mucosa

Blisters are localised pockets of fluid that form within or beneath the oral mucosa. Although blistering disorders are rare, symptoms can be very alarming

**Table 4.4** Blistering disorders of the oral mucosa.

| Type | Blister/disorder |
|------|------------------|
| Infective | Herpetic gingivostomatitis<br>Recurrent herpes simplex infection<br>Varicella zoster infection<br>Hand, foot and mouth disease<br>Herpangina |
| Autoimmune | Mucous membrane pemphigoid<br>Pemphigus<br>Linear IgA disease<br>Dermatitis herpetiformis |
| Others | Erythema multiforme<br>Angina bullosa haemorrhagica |

IgA, immunoglobulin A.

for patients and when severe with systemic involvement may require general medical care. The range of conditions that can present as blistering disorders is summarised in Table 4.4.

Although it is primarily a chronic mucocutaneous disorder, lichen planus can also present in an acute erosive form especially involving the buccal mucosa as illustrated in Figure 4.4. Mucous membrane pemphigoid primarily affects elderly females and gives rise to subepithelial bullae, painful erosions and mucosal scarring, which involving the eye may risk blindness. Pemphigus vulgaris is a rare condition affecting middle-aged females in which intra-epithelial vesicles and bullae form in the oral mucosa together with widespread skin involvement, which can be fatal without systemic treatment. In erythema multiforme, which often affects young adult males and may be drug-induced, systemic illness and fever is associated with swollen, bleeding and crusted lips together with erythema, ulceration and sloughing of the anterior oral mucosa.

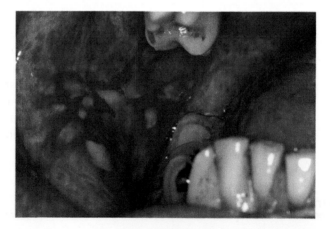

**Figure 4.4** Extensive erosive lichenoid lesion affecting buccal mucosa.

There is a range of other much rarer mucosal conditions such as epidermolysis bullosa, pyostomatitis vegetans, and linear IgA diseases together with oral hypersensitivity reactions to drugs all of which may give rise to vesicles, intra-epithelial abscesses and bulla formation, but their diagnosis and management lie outwith the remit of an emergency clinic. All suspected vesiculobullous disease patients should be referred for specialist oral medicine advice.

## Desquamative gingivitis

A particular clinical presentation of red and raw attached gingivae is termed desquamative gingivitis, and may be caused by erosive lichen planus, pemphigoid or pemphigus. This is usually easily distinguished from either an acute necrotising ulcerative gingivitis, in which anaerobic bacterial infection causes-crater shaped ulcers arising in interdental papillae, or primary herpetic gingivostomatitis in which there is diffuse erythema and oedema of the gingiva associated with widespread intra-oral vesicles and ulcers.

**Angina bullosa haemorrhagica** describes a specific condition, often seen in older patients, in which blood-filled blisters develop suddenly, usually on the soft palate or pharyngeal mucosa, giving rise to discomfort and dysphagia. The blisters breakdown and rupture after a day or two leaving ragged ulcerations, which eventually heal. There is no clear cause, although mucosal fragility with age and occasionally use of inhalers has been thought to be contributory. No treatment is particularly helpful and reassurance is usually all that is required. Repeated or persistent bouts of blistering should prompt referral to a specialist oral medicine clinic to rule out an underlying vesiculobullous disorder.

## Oral ulceration

Ulcers are full-thickness breaks in the continuity of oral mucosa, usually caused by death of epithelial cells, whilst erosions refer to areas of superficial epithelial tissue loss. A variety of mucosal disorders may present acutely as ulcerations and these are listed in Table 4.5. Definitive diagnosis and management

**Table 4.5** Causes of acute mucosal ulceration.

Trauma: Mechanical/thermal/chemical

Drug induced: Cytotoxics/nicorandil/NSAIDs

Recurrent aphthous stomatitis

Mucocutaneous disorders: Lichen planus/pemphigoid/pemphigus/erythema multiforme

Haematological disease: Anaemia/leukaemia

Malignancy: Squamous cell carcinoma/minor salivary gland carcinoma

NSAID, non-steroidal anti-inflammatory drug.

usually requires referral to oral medicine services but there are a series of important clinical observations every clinician should make when examining an ulcer (Box 4.2).

---

**Box 4.2   Examination of an ulcer**

- Define anatomical site
- Single or multiple
- Size (measure accurately)
- Shape – round/oval/irregular
- Base – soft/indurated/fixed
- Floor – smooth/granulating/sloughing/fungating
- Edge – distinct/raised/everted

---

Whilst multiple persistent ulcerations may represent mucocutaneous diseases such as pemphigoid or lichen planus, the most significant clinical presentation is, of course, the solitary non-healing ulcer present for longer than 2 weeks and which persists in the absence of an obvious traumatic cause. Here, one must consider oral squamous cell carcinoma as a possible cause. Classic signs of malignancy include irregular ulcer margins, raised or everted edges, induration (hardness) of the ulcer base and fixity to the surrounding tissues. Figure 4.5 illustrates the classical appearance of an invasive oral squamous cell carcinoma.

Oral cancer may present in a number of ways, however, and these are summarised in Box 4.3. It is also worth remembering that non-healing ulcerated or nodular lesions on the face, representing skin cancers such as basal cell carcinoma or squamous carcinoma may be noticed, often as incidental findings,

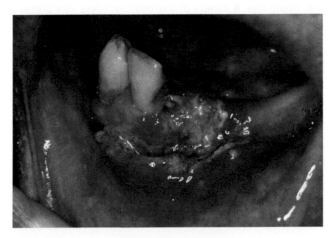

**Figure 4.5**   Invasive oral squamous cell carcinoma.

during oro-facial examination and practitioners should be alert to recognising and documenting such lesions during patient examination.

---

**Box 4.3    Clinical presentation of oral cancer**

- *Oral* ulceration (non-healing)
- *Red* or white patches
- *A*bnormal swellings
- *L*oss of tongue mobility
- *C*auliflower-like growths
- *A*bnormal, localised tooth mobility
- *N*on-healing tooth sockets
- *C*olour changes in mucosa (brown/blue)
- *E*rosions in mucosa
- *R*educed or altered sensation

---

An interesting, rare acute benign ulceration particularly affecting the tongue is the eosinophilic granuloma. Clinically, this tumour, like ulceration, may be mistaken for a squamous cell carcinoma but is usually a much softer lesion on palpation composed of eosinophils and histiocytes beneath the ulcerated mucosal surface. Whilst referral and biopsy for histopathological confirmation is mandatory, these lesions usually heal spontaneously within a few weeks, especially after an incisional biopsy that appears to stimulate the healing process.

Urgent referral to the local maxillofacial service is required for further assessment and management of all persistent or clinically suspicious ulcerated lesions.

## Disturbed oro-facial sensory or motor function

### Sensory changes

Acute onset of sensory disturbance in the trigeminal nerve distribution may be the result of traumatic injury, such as mental nerve anaesthesia following mandibular fracture or infra-orbital nerve paraesthesia after zygomatic fracture, but can also arise in infective conditions such as osteomyelitis.

Whilst many of these diagnoses can be confirmed on standard radiographic examination, the detailed assessment and management of sensory disturbance is better carried out in specialist oral medicine or maxillofacial clinics and patients with unexplained, persistent sensory loss should be referred for further investigation.

## Trismus

An acute onset of trismus, inability or limited ability to open the mouth, may represent an acute exacerbation of an underlying temporomandibular disorder, a submasseteric or pterygoid infection or, particularly in older patients, herald the presence of a previously occult squamous cell carcinoma arising in the retromolar and pterygoid regions.

In the event of suspicion, it is wise to refer such cases to an oral and maxillofacial surgeon for formal examination (often, under general anaesthesia) and head and neck imaging by computed tomography or magnetic resonance scanning.

## Facial palsy

Acute onset of facial paralysis is not uncommon in medical or surgical practice, but is less likely to present as a dental emergency. Nonethless, it is important that the dental practitioner has a clear understanding of the nature and presentation of this condition.

Facial nerve weakness may arise due to upper motor neurone lesions, such as a cerebrovascular accident, head injury or intra-cranial tumour, and gives rise to disturbed function in the lower part of the face only. These lesions preserve motor function to the forehead, which receives a bilateral innervation, and allows reactive facial expression with emotional response.

In contrast, lower motor neurone lesions arising from a Bell's palsy (nerve oedema in the facial nerve canal probably due to herpes virus infection), a malignant parotid gland or skull base tumour, or localised nerve trauma, produce total, ipsilateral facial weakness. Occasionally, a temporary facial palsy may follow administration of an inferior alveolar local analgesic injection during which diffusion of anaesthetic solution posteriorly through the parotid gland affects the main trunk of the facial nerve.

Patients sometimes present to dental clinics with a combination of trigeminal sensory nerve deficits together with facial nerve and other cranial nerve defects, and this usually suggests a more sinister underlying pathology such as a demyelinating disorder (multiple sclerosis) or a neoplastic process.

Patients presenting with persistent neurological symptoms should be referred to their medical practitioner or oral and maxillofacial surgery for further investigation and diagnosis.

## Haemorrhage

Whilst haemorrhage from the oro-facial region may present spontaneously, particularly from gingival tissue as a result of a bleeding diathesis or a haematological abnormality such as leukaemia, the most common cause is in response to trauma or a post-operative haemorrhage following dental extraction (see Chapter 11).

The history should help to determine the precise cause of a presenting haemorrhage, but a thorough and detailed clinical examination should be expedited to assess the patient's general condition, and pulse and blood pressure measurements should be taken to determine the risk of hypovolaemic shock. The management of an intra-oral haemorrhage is summarised in Box 4.4.

---

**Box 4.4    Management of Intra-oral haemorrhage**

- Review medical history and any recent surgery.
- Assess patient's general condition and measure pulse and blood pressure.
- Reassure patient and clean away excess blood.
- Careful oral examination in good light with adequate suction.
- Identify the precise source of bleeding.
- Administer local anaesthesia and apply pressure to wound for 10 minutes.
- Suture with or without packing of wound.
- Re-examine to confirm haemostasis.
- If persistent bleeding, refer to maxillofacial unit for specialist surgical management.

---

Any patient in whom haemorrhage fails to respond to appropriate local control measures should be referred urgently to oral and maxillofacial surgery for further investigation and management.

## Other acute conditions

### Immunodeficiency

Patients may be immunocompromised due to a number of factors, most commonly due to the long term use of immunosuppressive drugs following organ transplant but both congenital and acquired immunodeficiency states exist. Patients with HIV disease or AIDS may present with acute infective disorders such as florid candidosis, necrotising gingivitis and accelerated periodontitis, hairy leukoplakia (due to Epstein–Barr virus) or neoplastic disorders such as lymphoma or Kaposi's sarcoma. Once again, the patient's medical history and clinical examination should alert the clinician to the underlying cause and liaison with medical or infectious disease practitioners is mandatory.

### Facial soft tissue problems

Patients may present with acute infective conditions involving the facial skin such as erysipelas, impetigo or localised non-specific cellulitis. Similarly, acute sinus infections may give rise to facial and orbital swellings. Once a dental cause has been excluded, such patients are best referred to the maxillofacial unit for definitive management. This can be especially urgent for orbital swellings where untreated intra-orbital infection may endanger eyesight. Marked eyelid oedema and congestion, conjunctival redness and oedema, exophthalmos and pain are all signs requiring urgent surgical intervention.

Soft tissue abrasions and lacerations associated with facial or dentoalveolar fractures are commonly seen, as are the identification of foreign bodies, including tooth fragments, in the facial soft tissues. Whilst simple injuries may be treated in the emergency clinic, more extensive or complex soft tissue injuries should be referred for specialist maxillofacial surgery.

## Bony pathology

### Alveolar osteitis ('dry socket')

Post-extraction, if a blood clot forms inadequately in the socket or it is broken down, a painful osteitis may develop. This is often referred to as a 'dry socket'.
Pre-disposing factors to dry socket include the following:

- Smoking
- Surgical trauma
- Vasoconstrictor in local anaesthetic
- Oral contraceptives
- Mandibular tooth extractions
- History of radiotherapy or bisphosphonate medications (see later)

The principles of management are as follows:

- Irrigation of the socket (chlorhexidine or warmed saline to remove debris)
- Dressing the socket with bismuth iodoform paraffin paste and lidocaine gel on ribbon gauze to protect the socket from painful stimuli

#### Post-operative infection

If pus is seen in the socket and there is localised swelling and possibly lymphadenopathy, it has become infected and can often be managed as in dry socket, but usually antibiotics should be prescribed.

Practitioners should always consider why a socket has become infected. A radiograph is useful to see if there is a retained root or bony sequestrum. Clearly, if one or both is present, further treatment is indicated.

### Osteomyelitis

It is rare to see osteomyelitis in the jaws in most countries today. Radiographically, loss of the socket lamina dura will be seen with a rarefying osteitis in the bone. Sequestra may be seen. If caught early, osteomyelitis may be treated by antimicrobial therapy alone but often sequestrectomy is needed.

Osteoradionecrosis arises due to the death of irradiated and lethally damaged bone cells stimulated to divide following traumatic stimuli such as dental extractions or localised infection. Diminished vascularity of the periosteum also exists as a result of late radiation effects on endothelial lining cells, which is particularly pertinent for the dense and less vascular mandibular bone. The radionecrotic process usually starts as ulceration of the alveolar mucosa with brownish dead bone exposed at the base. Pathological fractures may occur in weakened bone and secondary infection leads to severe discomfort, trismus, foetor oris and general malaise. Radiographically, the earliest changes are a 'moth-eaten' appearance of the bone, followed by sequestration. All these potential complications should be considered in patients who have undergone radiotherapy of the head and neck, presenting at a dental emergency clinic.

Treatment should be predominately conservative, with long-term antibiotic and topical antiseptic therapy and careful local removal of sequestra when necessary. Hyperbaric oxygen and ultrasound therapy to increase tissue blood flow and oxygenation have also been recommended and are used as a treatment modality in the United Kingdom. It is best treated by a specialist in oral and maxillofacial surgery and prompt referral is important.

Osteonecrosis is a recently recognised complication of bisphosphonate treatment (Figure 4.6). This condition is defined as exposed bone in the maxillofacial region for longer than 8 weeks in the absence of radiotherapy but in a patient using bisphosphonates. It is diagnosed clinically but local malignancy must be excluded. Bisphosphonates are a group of drugs, including alendronic acid, disodium etidronate and risedronate sodium, which are adsorbed onto hydroxyapatite crystals, thus slowing their rate of growth and dissolution. They have been used in treatment of bony metastases, the hypercalcaemia of malignancy and the management of osteoporosis in post-menopausal women.

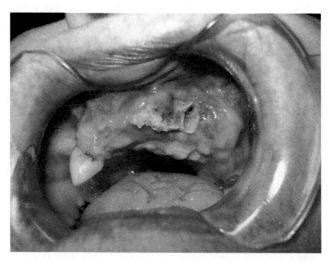

**Figure 4.6** Osteonecrosis following dental extractions.

Dental extractions should be avoided wherever possible while patients are on bisphosphonate therapy to reduce the risk of necrosis. Established cases require analgesia, long-term antibiotic and topical antiseptic therapy, together with careful local debridement to remove limited bony sequestra similar to the management of osteoradionecrosis. Risk factors that will increase the possibility of osteonecrosis developing include local infection, steroid use, trauma, chemotherapy and periodontal disease.

The mechanism by which bisphosphonates increase the risk of osteonecrosis is not fully understood. Trauma caused by a dental extraction in the presence of impaired osteoclast function may cause inadequate clearance of necrotic debris. Local osteonecrosis may also occur due to secondary infection. It is also thought that bisphosphonates might have toxic effects on soft tissues around the extraction site and thereby impair the function of vascular and epithelial cells.

Chemotherapy agents are inevitably highly toxic and risk important systemic effects such as infections and bleeding due to bone marrow involvement and resultant neutropaenia and thrombocytopaenia. It is important to liaise with an individual patient's oncologist to ensure dental or oral surgical treatments are timed to avoid periods of maximum bone marrow depression.

Management of established mucositis includes systemic analgesia, the use of intra-oral ice and topical analgesics such as benzydamine hydrochloride or 2% lidocaine lollipops or mouthwash.

Subsequent to radiotherapy and chemotherapy, meticulous oral hygiene is essential, especially during treatment when the mouth is inflamed and sore. Dilute chlorhexidine mouthwashes, topical fluoride applications, saliva substitutes and active restorative care may all be needed to preserve the remaining dentition. Should teeth have to be extracted, this is best carried out in a specialist oral and maxillofacial surgery unit and it is essential that atraumatic techniques are used, with primary closure of oral mucosa together with antibiotic therapy until healing is complete. Similar considerations apply to patients taking bisphosphonates. The timing of extractions in patients undergoing chemotherapy is critical. This should be coordinated with the treating oncologist so that the ideal 'window of opportunity' is used.

### Effects of drugs used in patients with oral malignancy on patient management in the dental emergency clinic

As mentioned previously, many drugs used in the management of malignant disease will affect white cell and platelet numbers. This means that bleeding and infection are risks of surgical dentistry such as extractions. A full blood count is needed to ensure that any extractions can be performed safely. Elective extractions should be carried out when the blood picture is normal, however, emergency extractions may need to be performed. If the platelet count is less than $50 \times 10^9$/L, then intra-oral surgery is contraindicated unless a platelet transfusion is provided; if less than $100 \times 10^9$/L, then sockets should be packed with a haemostatic agent such as Surgicel® and sutured. If the white cell count is less than $2.5 \times 10^9$/L, then prophylactic antibiotics are recommended.

It was mentioned previously that xerostomia and stomatitis are side effects of radiotherapy. These can also be unwanted effects of some drugs used to treat malignancy. Thus, excellent oral hygiene and caries prevention measures such as the use of fluoride are recommended. If dentures are ill-fitting, these should be removed as they may worsen drug-induced mucositis.

Some of the drugs used to treat malignancies will interfere with medications dentists might prescribe. Examples include paracetamol and metronidazole, both of which increase the toxicity of busulphan by inhibiting metabolism and increasing plasma concentration of the cytotoxic drug. Similarly, erythromycin increases the toxicity of the chemotherapeutic drug vinblastine. The toxicity of methotrexate is increased with concomitant administration of non-steroidal anti-inflammatory drugs, penicillins and tetracyclines. These are just some examples of pertinent drug interactions. The dental surgeon should consult a publication such as the *British National Formulary* or discuss with the patient's oncologist.

## Summary

It is clear that many oral diseases may present in the dental emergency clinic presenting as a myriad of fascinating oral surgery and oral medical conditions. The emergency clinic practitioner's role, however, is not one of specialist diagnosis and management but rather the recognition of those important and/or life-threatening disorders that require referral. Indeed, a close and harmonious working relationship between the dental emergency clinic and their local departments of oral and maxillofacial surgery and oral medicine is imperative for appropriate, comprehensive and efficacious patient care.

## Further reading

Meechan JG, Greenwood M, Moore UJ, Thomson PJ, Brook IM, Smith KG (2006) *Minor Oral Surgery in Dental Practice*. Quintessence Publishing Co Ltd, London.
Moore UJ (ed.) (2011) *Principles of Oral and Maxillofacial Surgery* (6th edition). Blackwell Science, Oxford.
Scully C (2004) *Oral and Maxillofacial Medicine*. Wright, Edinburgh.

# Chapter 5
# Restorative Dental Emergencies

## A. Moufti and C.B. Hayward

## Introduction

Dental surgeons working in dental emergency clinics will encounter dental emergencies on a daily basis. Most of these emergencies usually require some form of restorative care. This chapter covers the diagnosis and management of common conditions requiring emergency restorative care.

Broadly speaking, patients who seek dental emergency care usually complain of pain, swelling(s) and problems with the structural integrity and retention of teeth, fillings and prostheses. One study of patient attendance for emergency care in a British dental teaching hospital showed that most patients complained of oro-facial pain (77%), swelling (22%) or a lost restoration (21%) (Scully, 1995). Another, community-based study reported that pain and prosthetic problems were the most frequent reasons for consulting an emergency dental hospital department in France (34% and 42% retrospectively) (Roger-Leroi et al, 2007).

It is essential that the clinician is able to correctly diagnose the presenting condition and carry out effective emergency care in an expeditious manner. It is equally important that every dental emergency clinic adopts a policy for management of emergency walk-in patients or telephone calls. The use of a triage system is invaluable in managing these cases efficiently. Various questionnaires and decision-making 'trees' are available to reach sound diagnoses and management decisions. Table 5.1 gives an overview of many conditions requiring emergency or urgent restorative care.

This chapter cannot cover every possible situation that could arise but addresses the more common conditions that may present. In view of this, it is important that certain basic principles are adhered to for safe patient management.

*Dental Emergencies*, First Edition. Edited by Mark Greenwood and Ian Corbett.
© 2012 Blackwell Publishing Ltd. Published 2012 by Blackwell Publishing Ltd.

**Table 5.1** Summary of most common reasons for seeking emergency restorative care.

| Presenting complaint | Structure involved | Condition | Causes |
|---|---|---|---|
| Pain | Tooth (pulp) | Sensitivity<br>Pulpitis | Caries<br>Crack or fracture<br>Wear (abrasion, attrition, erosion and abfraction)<br>Failing restoration<br>Gingival recession<br>Iatrogenic, e.g. scaling, whitening, over-preparation, overload, galvanic pain, composite shrinkage |
| | Periodontium | Acute gingivitis and periodontitis<br>Abscesses<br>ANUG | Infection (periodontal or pulpal)<br>Trauma, e.g. occlusion, impacted food and foreign bodies<br>Iatrogenic, e.g. over-instrumentation of root canals or root surface, overhangs, impinging denture clasp |
| | Mucosa | Stomatitis | Infection-related[a]<br>Prosthesis-related, e.g. ill-fitting denture[a] |
| | Bone | For example, inflammatory bony conditions | |
| | Other | Referred pain from another tooth or structure<br>Neurological, e.g. Trigeminal nerve neuralgia[a]<br>Psychologic pain, e.g. atypical facial pain[a] | |
| Swelling | Mucosa[a] | Periapical or periodontal abscess | Infection |
| Tooth structural integrity (cracks, fractures, and mobility) | Tooth | Chipping<br>Cracked tooth syndrome<br>Fracture | Trauma (impact or occlusal)<br>Caries<br>Internal resorption<br>Over-preparation |

**Table 5.1** (*Continued*)

| Presenting complaint | Structure involved | Condition | Causes |
|---|---|---|---|
| | Fillings Prosthesis | Loosening, debonding, decementation Fracture | Marginal leakage Caries Construction errors |
| | Periodontal | Dislocation and avulsion Loss of attachment | Trauma (impact or occlusal) Periodontal disease |
| | Bone[a] | Fracture Bone loss | Trauma Pathology, e.g. cysts, neoplasms |

ANUG, acute necrotising ulcerative gingivitis.
[a]Consult the relevant chapter for differential diagnosis.

## General principles

The aetiology and management of restorative dental emergencies is usually relatively straightforward. More serious conditions can present on occasion with similar clinical presentations. It is for this reason in particular that the practitioner should carry out a thorough work up.

All patients should have a thorough history taken, along the lines discussed in Chapter 2.

A thorough clinical examination should be carried out, looking for any teeth that are sensitive to percussion. In addition, tooth mobility, periodontal pocketing, caries, soft tissue swelling, fractures, the condition of existing restorations and pulp vitality should all be borne in mind. Appropriate special tests should be obtained according to accepted criteria and must potentially influence patient management to be fully justified.

## Pain management

Dental pain, ranging from tooth sensitivity to throbbing, intractable pain, comprises around 20–75% of reasons for seeking emergency dental care. A summary is given in Table 5.2.

### Dentine hypersensitivity

Dentine hypersensitivity is defined as a short, sharp pain that arises from exposed dentine in response to a stimulus, commonly cold, hot, evaporative, tactile, osmotic or chemical that cannot be attributed to any other dental cause. It is a diagnosis of exclusion. Prevalence is variable but has been

**Table 5.2** Summary of common dental pain conditions requiring emergency restorative care.

| | Reversible pulpitis | Irreversible pulpitis | Acute apical periodontitis | Acute apical abscess | Acute periodontal abscess | Dentine hypersensitivity | Food packing | Cracked tooth syndrome | Chronic apical periodontitis |
|---|---|---|---|---|---|---|---|---|---|
| Points in the history | Short, sharp pain, well localised, mainly with cold, goes when stimulus removed | Rapid onset of pain, can be spontaneous, poorly localised, can be referred to opposing or adjacent teeth persists after stimulus removed Sleep disturbed | Constant pain, particularly on biting, occurred over short time Can be throbbing in nature Rarely sensitive to thermal change | Rapid onset of pain, variable intensity, throbbing Pain on biting well localised | Localised swelling some pain | Pain with hot, cold and sweet | Pain after eating fibrous foods | Sharp pain on biting and with hot and cold fluids Pain on release of pressure Absence of sensitivity to heat Long history of symptoms | Pain in the past, now no longer sensitive to hot and cold |
| Findings on clinical examination | Caries, recent filling, failing restoration | Extensive caries, failed restoration, endodontic treatment | Swelling palpable but localised to tooth, tooth may be tender over the apex | Swelling palpable and fluctuant, can be intra- or extra-oral | Intra-oral swelling adjacent to tooth at gingival margin Increased tooth mobility | Gingival recession, failing restoration margins, exposed dentine Exclusion of all other causes | Lost or broken contact point(s). Gingival inflammation, food debris often caught in the failed contact point | Fracture line may be evident | Large restoration or caries |

| | Reversible pulpitis | Irreversible pulpitis | Acute apical periodontitis | Acute apical abscess | Acute periodontal abscess | Dentine hypersensitivity | Food packing | Cracked tooth syndrome | Chronic apical periodontitis |
|---|---|---|---|---|---|---|---|---|---|
| Vitality tests | Positive with cold, increased response to electrical pulp tester | Hyperalgesic pulp, more intensely responsive to cold stimulation, persists after removal of stimulus Later, cold may ease pain | Negative vitality or delayed response | Negative | Often positive | Positive | Positive/negative vitality | Positive vitality exaggerated response to cold thermal challenge | Negative vitality |
| Findings on percussion | Not TTP | TTP | TTP | TTP and tender to touch | Slight tenderness but in a more lateral than apical direction | Not TTP | Not TTP can be tender on lateral percussion | TTP on occasions | TTP may sound dull on percussion |
| Other clinical findings | | Pain can be spontaneous Pain if mechanical, chemo or thermal stimulation from food entering cavity | | Pyrexia, malaise | Deep pocketing, pus released on probing | | No resistance to floss passing through contact point | Pain on release of pressure on opening from compression with cotton roll. Pain lateral pressure onto cusp with 'tooth sleuth'® | |

**Table 5.2** (Continued).

| | Reversible pulpitis | Irreversible pulpitis | Acute apical periodontitis | Acute apical abscess | Acute periodontal abscess | Dentine hypersensitivity | Food packing | Cracked tooth syndrome | Chronic apical periodontitis |
|---|---|---|---|---|---|---|---|---|---|
| Radiographic examination | Superficial caries or cavity penetration Lamina dura seen no apical change | Extensive caries involving the pulp, either primary or secondary under a restoration Widening of PMS Usually, no periapical change | Usually, no radiographic changes, occasionally, widening of PMS | No findings to large periapical lucency | No periapical changes except in a perio-endo lesion Alveolar bone loss can be vertical or horizontal | May be some alveolar bone loss | None or may see alveolar bone loss - vertical and/or horizontal | None | Periapical radiolucency |
| Findings on investigation | Caries, recent filling, failing restoration | Necrotic pulp | Necrotic pulp | Pus may drain from root canal | | Recent tooth scaling or root planing, tooth whitening, periodontal disease | | Crack may be visible in the base after removal of an existing restoration Crack might be seen in enamel Staining in the enamel crack, clicking felt when running the probe over the enamel surface | Necrotic pulp |

TTP, tender to percussion; PMS, periodontal membrane space.

estimated to be between 4% and 57%. However, in patients with periodontitis, it can be as high as 60–80%. Dentine hypersensitivity presents as a severe problem in 1% of patients.

Distribution occurs mostly in the 30–40 year age group and is more common in women than men. Any age group and any tooth can be affected. It commonly arises at the cervical margins on the labial and buccal tooth surfaces. Not all exposed dentine surfaces are sensitive. Sensitivity is initiated when the smear layer has been removed, opening the dentinal tubules. Tooth substance loss due to erosion and attrition may also be implicated.

Following a correct diagnosis, treatment follows two distinct pathways, in-surgery treatment and home treatment, followed by review should the condition not resolve.

In-surgery treatments include topically applied desensitising agents such as fluoride as sodium or stannous fluoride. Potassium nitrate can be applied topically as a gel or aqueous solution. Sealants in the form of adhesive resins applied to the areas of sensitive dentine to occlude open tubules may be used.

Other less commonly used or accessible treatments include: iontophoresis in conjunction with fluoride pastes. Laser treatment has been employed in some cases (Nd:YAG). In-home treatment includes improved oral hygiene techniques and the use of non-abrasive dentifrices, the use of desensitising toothpastes and fluoride mouthwashes.

## Reversible pulpitis

Reversible pulpitis presents as summarised below:

- Pain with hot, cold and sweet.
- Pain is short and sharp, mediated by the A delta fibres (see Chapter 8).
- Pain that ceases when the stimulus is removed. Can be difficult to locate.
- Electric pulp test (EPT) within normal limits but can be hyperalgesic.
- Percussion test within normal limits. There will be pain if dentine is cut.
- Radiographs may show caries or an extensive restoration.

### Management
- Check the occlusion and remove non-working facets.
- Caries removal where appropriate and place a sedative dressing. This may be a calcium hydroxide (setting) liner and glass ionomer cement (GIC) placed to provide an effective seal.
- Advise to attend for further assessment of restorative needs and definitive treatment.

## Irreversible pulpitis

- Pain with hot, cold and sweet stimuli.
- Pain is persistent, C fibre pain. Lasts minutes or hours after the stimulus has been removed.

- Pain is spontaneous, throbbing in character, can disturb sleep, is often difficult to localise, eased with analgesics.
- In advanced cases, cold can ease the pain and heat will make it worse.
- EPT is not helpful in early cases. Can be within normal limits, the responses can be variable, delayed or early.
- There is no pain if the dentine is cut if the coronal pulp is non-vital.
- Percussion tests are within normal limits.
- Radiographs may show deep caries or large restorations and occasionally early widening of the apical periodontal membrane space.

### Management

Ideal treatment consists in accessing the pulp chamber and the complete extirpation of the coronal and radicular pulp. This should be carried out under the cover of rubber dam. The pulp should be completely removed from the root(s) and pulp chamber, the root canals measured for working length, the root canal(s) shaped and cleaned using a solution of sodium hypochlorite at a dilution between 0.5% and 5%. The pulp chamber and root canal(s) should then be dried and sealed with a dry sterile cotton wool pledget and the tooth sealed with a dressing using GIC. The danger if the procedure is incompletely performed is laceration of the pulp contents, its incomplete removal resulting in further pain and the possible introduction of sepsis. At the least it would create difficulties for the subsequent treatment and in particular the successful use of local anaesthesia, due to increased pulpal inflammation.

An alternative treatment modality is to remove the coronal pulp and the coronal portions of the radicular pulp, irrigation with chlorhexidine solution and the placement of an antibiotic or corticosteroid dressing on a cotton wool pledget with the introduction of the dressing material into the coronal portion of the root canal system. A guide to which treatment to use is to look for the top of the radicular pulps and if there are bleeding surfaces, then it would be reasonable to use this compromise system. If there is still necrotic tissue within the root canals, then the canals should be accessed as first described.

Post-treatment pain may be due to several different causes:

- The tooth may be over-filled and 'high' in the bite.
- Laceration of vital pulp tissue, incomplete extirpation, over-instrumentation and trauma to the periapical tissues.
- Inadvertent extrusion of sodium hypochlorite solution into the periapical tissues.
- Perforation of the root or coronal walls.
- Unrecognised aberrant root canal.

It is essential that the root canal system is effectively sealed to prevent contamination and/or re-infection. If pain persists after initial treatment, then further irrigation of the root canal system and perhaps further instrumentation will be required, accompanied by further irrigation with hypochlorite solution or chlorhexidine solution.

## Infections and soft tissue problems

### Acute periapical abscess

Irreversible pulpitis progresses to an acute apical periodontitis and then to acute periapical periodontitis (Figures 5.1 and 5.2). This is a dynamic change and in the early stages of each condition a differential diagnosis can be difficult to elucidate. There are changes in the radiographic appearance, from a slight widening of the periodontal membrane shadow to a well-marked area. The tooth will become very tender and may show extrusion from the socket with increasing mobility. There will be an associated soft tissue swelling. The tooth will be non-vital. This is very important in the differential diagnosis between an acute apical abscess (non-vital) and a lateral periodontal abscess in which the pulp will usually be vital on testing.

#### Management
Drainage is the key, initially by opening up the root canal system and allowing drainage 'through' the tooth. The resulting drop in pressure will ease the

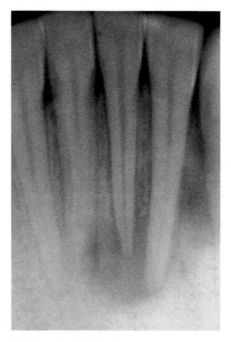

**Figure 5.1** Periapical view showing an extensive area of rarefaction at the apices of 31, 32. This lesion was associated with a sinus draining through the skin covering the chin.

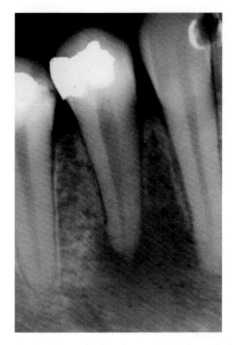

**Figure 5.2** Periapical radiograph showing periapical rarefaction in a case of acute apical periodontitis.

pain. In the presence of an intra-oral swelling that is fluctuant, drainage may need to be established by incision. A large extra-oral swelling or a spreading cellulitis in the neck associated with pyrexia and dysphagia requires referral to a department of oral and maxillofacial surgery for urgent treatment as the condition can rapidly become life-threatening.

Local anaesthesia can be difficult to achieve by local infiltration and a regional nerve block may be more successful.

## Acute periodontal abscess

A periodontal abscess is an acute, destructive process in the periodontium that results in the localised collection of pus communicating with the oral cavity through the gingival sulcus or other periodontal sites not arising from the tooth pulp.

### Aetiology

Cases of acute periodontal abscess tend to occur in a pre-existing periodontal pocket. If drainage through the pocket is blocked, then there is a build up of pus. This results in the recognisable clinical signs. Periodontal abscesses can also occur following professional mechanical tooth cleaning if there is inadequate instrumentation of the base of the periodontal pocket or furcation area.

A compromised immune response may predispose a patient to periodontal pocket formation. Multiple periodontal abscesses are seen typically in poorly controlled diabetic patients, for example.

### Clinical features

Pain, oedema and erythema of the involved periodontal tissues may all be seen. If there is systemic involvement, lymphadenopathy or lymphadenitis may be detected. The tooth involved is tender to the bite and tender to percussion. Periodontal pocketing is usually found, the tooth might be extruded slightly from its socket and a discharging sinus may be evident.

### Diagnosis

Diagnosis of periodontal abscess is from the history and examination. Radiographs are helpful in confirming the diagnosis; commonly a radiolucency in the lateral aspect of the periodontium is seen. If the infection is sited on either the buccal, palatal or lingual aspect, little radiographic evidence may be seen.

### Differential diagnosis

Differential diagnosis must be made between an acute apical periodontitis and an acute periodontal abscess as there are similar signs and symptoms in both conditions. They differ in that a tooth with an acute periodontal abscess often is vital and is painful to lateral percussion. A tooth with an acute apical periodontitis is usually non-vital and tender to vertical percussion. Radiographic changes are seen apically. Conversely, the radiographic changes, if seen, are lateral in the periodontal membrane space in a periodontal abscess. A sinus, if present, is found near the tooth apex in the case of acute periodontitis, and between the apex and the gingival margin in the case of acute periodontal abscess. Drainage and antibiotic therapy are the mainstays of treatment.

### Treatment of a gingival abscess or an acute periodontal abscess

The dental surgeon should give a local anaesthetic, establish drainage and debride the lesion. In the case of a gingival abscess, blade incision is used to establish drainage. Drainage for the periodontal abscess is achieved with an external incision or by curette via the pocket. Care should be taken not to over-instrument the root surface as this decreases the prospects for reattachment. After drainage is established, the area should be irrigated with warm saline solution or water. For a periodontal abscess, antibiotics should be prescribed if the patient is experiencing malaise, lymphadenopathy or is febrile. Analgesics may be prescribed for pain. After treatment of an acute abscess, the patient should return the next day. The clinician should evaluate the area, to assess the need for further treatment (such as surgery) after the acute symptoms have resolved.

## Acute gingivitis

Gingivitis can be defined as inflammation of the gingivae. This is caused by a build up of plaque. Plaque is a biofilm formed on the tooth surface consisting of oral bacteria (*Streptococcus*, *Actinomyces*, gram-positive and gram-negative anaerobic rods) that are embedded in a polymer matrix of bacterial and salivary origin. Plaque forms a layer over the surfaces of the gums and teeth in stagnant and protected surfaces. The bacteria in plaque release toxins, enzymes and metabolic products that cause local inflammation and damage to the gingivae; hence, gingival bleeding particularly on toothbrushing is one of the signs of gingivitis. The removal or inhibition of microbial plaque can prevent development of gingivitis.

A large proportion of the population (70–90% of the adult population), is estimated to have some degree of gingivitis. Gingivitis is more prevalent in older adults, although it can be found at any age after tooth eruption.

Treatment of gingivitis takes three forms:

(1) Physical removal of plaque by efficient toothbrushing, or professional mechanical tooth cleaning.
(2) Chemical inhibition of bacterial plaque formation using mouthwashes containing chlorhexidine solution.
(3) Dental health education and oral hygiene instruction to correct deficiencies in cleaning techniques are important.

Clearly, management can only be initiated in the dental emergency clinic and patients require careful follow-up by the patients' regular practitioner.

## Acute periodontitis

Periodontitis is a sequel to untreated gingivitis. It is characterised by inflammation and loss of bone support for the tooth and the breakdown of the periodontal attachment. The teeth become less securely attached and untreated periodontitis carries a risk of tooth loss. People with diabetes may have an above-average chance of developing periodontitis.

If gingivitis is prevented or treated, the development of periodontitis is prevented.

### Complications of gingivitis

The symptoms of mild gingival disease are bleeding gums and halitosis. This may progress to spontaneous bleeding with loss of bone, periodontal attachment loss and eventual tooth loss. There is also the risk of localised infection within the periodontal membrane – a periodontal abscess.

There are also more serious potential consequences. The barrier function of the gingival tissue is reduced in people with gingivitis. This means that toxins and bacteria may enter the bloodstream through the gingivae. The implications of this can be serious:

- Dental plaque bacteria, after entering the bloodstream, can become trapped in atheromatous plaques within the arteries. People with severe periodontal disease are possibly more likely to have an acute myocardial infarction or a stroke than those without it.
- Patients with lung conditions may find that periodontal disease increases their chance of a respiratory tract infection.
- Periodontal disease in pregnancy is possibly a predictor of low birth weight, as plaque bacteria are thought to produce cervical/uterine inflammation and therefore premature birth.

In summary, there are strong arguments for the treatment and prevention of gingival disease, for reasons beyond purely dental health – particularly in high-risk groups.

### Gingival problems and dental implants

With the increasing number of patients with dental implants, the dental surgeon should always consider the possibility of having to manage inflammation in the periodontal tissues around an implant.

Most inflammatory conditions relating to implants can be corrected with attention to oral hygiene and professional cleaning. Although the management principles are the same, some differences exist. For example, calculus should be removed from titanium abutments with instruments that will not damage the surface of the implant. Ultrasonic instruments and steel-tipped instruments are contraindicated.

Furthermore, when investigating a case of periodontitis around implants, attention should be paid to some specific potential causes. These include loosening or ill-adaption of the crown above the implant leading to marginal leakage. The clinician also needs to ensure there is no cement residue that is extruded from the implant/crown joint.

### Acute necrotising ulcerative gingivitis

Acute necrotising ulcerative gingivitis (ANUG) is acute inflammation of the gingivae that is characterised by painful swelling, formation of ulcers and the sloughing of necrotic tissue, commonly seen at the interdental papillae. The pain can be intense and is often associated with pyrexia and characteristic foetor. The organisms involved are commonly *Prevotella intermedia*, alpha-haemolytic streptococci, *Actinomyces* species and spirochaetes.

The aim of treatment is to provide relief of pain and sepsis. This is achieved by an initial scaling to remove necrotic debris and calculus, although a more thorough scaling will be required at a subsequent appointment. The scaling should be accompanied by irrigation of the gingival tissues with a solution of chlorhexidine. In severe cases, where there is systemic involvement, antibiotics should be prescribed, such as metronidazole. Amoxicillin could be used if metronidazole is inappropriate. A mouthwash of chlorhexidine solution should be advised. An alternative would be a 6% hydrogen peroxide mouthwash, marketed as Bocasan®. Analgesics such as paracetamol or ibuprofen should be advised.

Noma (cancrum oris) is a condition in which ANUG spreads beyond the gingivae to involve the mouth and face. This condition is rarely seen in the developed world.

## Stomatitis

Stomatitis is inflammation of the lining of any of the soft tissue structures in the mouth. The causes range from infective (bacterial, viral or fungal), inflammatory, traumatic, environmental, neoplastic, idiopathic, degenerative or congenital. The scope of this chapter is limited and the following are some of the more common conditions encountered where the restorative situation may be related. More detail can be found in Chapter 4.

## Denture stomatitis (chronic atrophic candidosis)

Chronic atrophic candidosis is a common condition found in around 50% of denture wearers. It is more commonly found in the elderly and those living in nursing homes than the young. This is a condition that can often be regarded as a secondary candidal infection of tissues modified by the wearing of dentures. Often, these patients will wear the denture 24 hours per day and do not maintain an adequate degree of denture hygiene. The dentures are frequently ill-fitting. The denture-bearing area is chronically erythematous and oedematous. It is more commonly seen under the upper denture.

### Management
The patient is advised to reduce the amount of time the dentures are worn in any 24-hour-period to a minimum, in particular to leave them out at night when in bed. This may cause a lot of social difficulty for a patient and the advising surgeon should be practical with this advice to allow the patient a degree of control in this part of the treatment. If the patient is 'over-directed', there may be a lack of compliance and the condition will persist. The denture should be cleaned and soaked overnight in either a weak hypochlorite solution or chlorhexidine. Hypochlorite should not be used with metal-based dentures as this will cause staining.

### Antifungal treatment
If the condition does not resolve, or if fungal organisms are identified, antifungal treatment is indicated. Topical treatment is often the first-line therapy. Clotrimazole cream may be applied to the fitting surface of the denture and the denture refitted. Fluconazole may be indicated.

In some cases, where the condition fails to respond to treatment, a systemic disease may be producing an impact on the oral mucosa. Commonly, type

2 diabetes, other conditions include immunodeficiency disorders, HIV or antibiotic therapy.

## Angular cheilitis

Angular cheilitis is an inflammatory condition characterised by deep cracks or splits at the commissures of the mouth. It often occurs bilaterally. The splits are painful and may bleed when the mouth is opened. There may be formation of a crust or ulcer in the area. These areas are susceptible to infection with *Candida albicans* or other pathogens such as staphylococci. The condition is often found in the elderly or others who have decreased vertical dimension either from the loss of teeth or ill-fitting dentures.

Angular cheilitis is also associated with nutritional deficiencies and iron deficiency anaemia, zinc deficiency, poor diet and medications that can dry the skin.

## Traumatic soft tissue lesions

Soft tissue trauma may occur as a result of ill-fitting prostheses, sharp teeth or restorations, cheek biting, parafunctional habits or thermal burns. The diagnosis will usually become evident from the history and examination. Treatment usually consists of removing the traumatic cause, adjusting or replacing prostheses or fillings and teeth where needed, the prevention of parafunctional habits and advice and analgesics in the case of thermal burns.

## Crack, fracture and mobility of teeth and dental restorations

Crack, fracture and mobility of a tooth, or part of it, are all interlinked and are best described together. For example, the pain experienced from a cracked tooth is not dissimilar to that from a fractured root. Furthermore, mobility might be the only clinical manifestation of a fractured tooth.

A complaint of tooth mobility is common and has a wide variety of causes. To facilitate a differential diagnosis, Table 5.3 divides these problems into two major groups: supra-gingival and sub-gingival. However, the clinician should be fully aware of the strong interlink between these, and the potential similarity in presentation. Differential diagnosis relies on a sound history and clinical examination, for example, using digital manipulation and percussion; as well as other investigations, especially radiographs taken from different angles.

Although a mobile tooth may not initially be perceived as an emergency, it should be investigated thoroughly and addressed promptly, as the consequences can be costly and even life-threatening should a bone neoplasm be misdiagnosed, or delay of recementation of a mobile crown, which can then be inhaled or ingested.

Regardless of the case or cause, it is of paramount importance that the clinician checks occlusion both in inter-cuspal position (ICP) and guidance to

**Table 5.3** Most common reasons for tooth mobility.

| Mobility level | Problem | Reason | Investigation | Management |
|---|---|---|---|---|
| Supra-gingival | Loose/fractured filling or part of the tooth crown | • Underlying caries<br>• Trauma (impact or occlusal) | | |
| | Loose crown/retainer | Crown:<br>• Fracture<br>• Decementation (or loosening of the crown retention screw on an implant)<br>Foundation:<br>• Fracture of the abutment<br>• Fracture/decementation of a post | | |
| Sub-gingival | Vertical or horizontal root fracture | • Occlusal trauma<br>• Impact trauma<br>• Internal resorbtion<br>• Over-preparation (perforation or use of a large post) | | |
| | Tooth dislocation | • Impact trauma | | Splint |
| | Mobility associated with loss of bone support | • Advanced periodontal disease<br>• Occlusal trauma<br>• Underlying bone pathology, e.g. cysts, neoplasms | Periapical X-ray | Perio therapy<br>Occlusal adjustment |

ensure there is no overload on the tooth involved in the fracture or mobility. Occasionally, there may be a need for a complete alleviation of occlusal contacts in ICP in the case of excruciating pain.

## Tooth cracks, fractures and mobility

Tooth fracture and avulsion caused by trauma are covered in Chapter 7.

## The 'cracked tooth syndrome'

Tooth crack is an incomplete fracture of enamel or dentine and therefore is not usually associated with noticeable mobility. It can be caused by excessive force applied to a healthy tooth or physiologic forces applied to a weakened tooth. Causes of cracks are numerous.

Teeth most commonly involved tend to be lower molars, followed by upper premolars and molars, while mandibular premolars are the least affected. The condition is most common in patients at the age range of 30-60 years. A summary of the most common reasons for cracked tooth syndrome is given in Box 5.1.

### Diagnosis

The diagnosis of cracked tooth is often difficult. A careful history and assessment of the symptoms, in particular that of cold sensitivity and sharp pain on biting hard or tough food, which starts on the release of pressure, is an important indicator. Symptoms may vary according to the depth and orientation of the crack.

### Investigations

(1) During visual inspection, the use of magnifying loupes and transillumination with the aid of a fibre-optic device may be helpful.
(2) The use of a sharp straight probe may also help detect 'catches' in the cracks.
(3) The removal of existing restorations may also help to reveal fracture lines.
(4) The use of stains to highlight fracture lines such as gentian violet or methylene blue.
(5) The use of the so-called bite tests to mimic the symptoms associated with incomplete fractures of posterior teeth. However, it is important to gain prior consent from the patient as the use of such a test may cause cuspal fragmentation. Examples of these are 'Fractfinder (Denbur, Oak Brook, IL, USA) and 'Tooth sleuth II®'.
(6) Vitality tests for involved teeth are usually positive, although sometimes affected teeth may display signs of hypersensitivity to cold thermal stimuli due to the presence of pulpal inflammation.
(7) Radiographs tend to be of limited use, as fractures tend to propagate in a mesiodistal direction, parallel to that of the plane of the film.

**Box 5.1 Summary of most common reasons for cracked tooth syndrome**

*Iatrogenic*
- Excessive removal of tooth tissue during cavity preparation
- Placement of poor-quality dental amalgam alloys
- Over-contouring of restorations
- Placement of 'friction lock' or 'self-threading dentine pins'
- The non-incremental application of composite resin
- Excessive hydraulic pressure when luting inlays, onlays or crowns

*Occlusal factors*
- Masticatory accident, e.g. biting suddenly on a hard object such as bone with excessive force. Other commonly attributing food items/objects include betel nut chewing, inadvertent biting of lead shot, cherry stones and 'granary' bread
- Parafunctional tooth grinding habits, in particular the habit of nocturnal bruxism
- The loss of anterior guidance, which may lead to the generation of harmful eccentric forces

*Developmental*
- Areas of localised structural weakness within a tooth as a result of incomplete fusion of areas of calcification
- Morphological features including deep occlusal grooves, pronounced vertical radicular grooves or bifurcations, extensive pulp spaces, steep cusp angles, prominent mesio-palatal cusps of upper first molars and the presence of lingually inclined mandibular molar teeth

*Others*
- The effect of lingual barbells, erosive tooth wear and the factor of thermal cycling, which may induce enamel cracks
- An ageing dentition as dental hard tissues become more brittle and less elastic with age

**Emergency treatment for 'cracked tooth syndrome'**

Aim of treatment is to prevent crack propagation and to relieve the associated symptoms.

### Treatment options

(1) *Occlusal adjustment*: This can be done by grinding the tooth out of occlusion. However, this approach is of limited benefit as the tooth may still be critically stressed by a food bolus. Furthermore, occlusal adjustment may not only involve the removal of healthy sound tooth tissue, but when undertaken without analysing the effects on the residual dentition may also lead to unwanted occlusal interferences elsewhere in the dental arch.

(2) *Removal of a pre-existing restoration*: This should be done to assess the full extent of the fracture.

(3) *Immobilisation of segment*: An extra-coronal circumferential splint may be applied. This may take the form of a copper ring or a stainless steel orthodontic band. However, this may be time consuming and technically challenging. In addition, patients may object to the aesthetics where the band is visible.

(4) *Direct composite splint*: This can be used with minimal tooth reduction of the functional areas of the occlusal surface or a non-invasive splint with no tooth reduction, creating a flat splint in a supra-occlusal position. Resin composite is applied to a thickness of 1.0–1.5 mm over the occlusal surface of the affected tooth.

## Fracture and mobility of restorations

Patients with ditched, fractured, dislodged or lost fillings may complain of pain or sharp edges, as well as the aesthetic consequences if the filling in question is readily visible. The pain symptoms, caused by dentine exposure underneath the filling, could present as hypersensitivity, pulpitis or even as periodontal/periapical abscess symptoms in advanced cases. Sharp edges could often result in irritation to the side of tongue or the cheek potentially leading to an ulcer.

Restorative materials today have low failure rates. Survival rates are reported around 93% after 7 years for amalgam and composite, while gold and ceramic fillings have higher longevity. However, the longevity of restorations is undoubtedly influenced by the operator, the patient and the material. Therefore, it is important to undertake a careful investigation into the cause of pain under fillings in order to establish a sound differential diagnosis. Differential diagnosis for pain following filling placement should include cavity over-preparation, material (composite) shrinkage and occlusal trauma.

Examination should include the marginal integrity, fracture line and potential extension to the tooth substance and the presence of secondary caries. Any dental examination should also include a check for occlusal load (in ICP) and guidance. It is also very important that the dentist examines the cavity design for retention and resistance to avoid future fracture and dislodgement.

Additional investigation may also include vitality testing, transillumination (see Section 'The Cracked Tooth Syndrome') as well as radiographs.

## Emergency management

Pain management depends on the diagnosis, and the reader is referred to Section 'Pain management'. Sharp edges can easily be dealt with smoothing of the filling or tooth edges.

The choice of material for emergency replacement of lost or fractured filling depends on a number of factors, including the following:

- *The position and visibility*:The clinician needs to make a judgement between replacing a fractured composite filling with composite or patching it temporarily with GIC.
- *The material*: A chairside replacement of a porcelain or gold filling is unlikely to be possible. Therefore, the filling should be removed and replaced by another temporarily. Alternatively, temporary patching with composite can be undertaken (see Section 'Fracture of the porcelain veneers or a porcelain-fused-to-metal crown').
- *The tooth prognosis*: Including tooth's vitality and restorability, and the need for root canal treatment or crowning.

Having placed a temporary filling, the operator should check and adjust its occlusion.

## Fracture and mobility of fixed prostheses

It is not uncommon to see patients with loose or dislodged crowns or bridges. The majority of these are usually temporary crowns. The consequences of a crown becoming loose could be problematic, including the risk of ingestion and less likely, inhalation.

Patients with loose crowns usually complain of dental hypersensitivity, adverse appearance as well as the worry of a sudden dislodgement and swallowing of the loose crown. Some will also report gingivitis or a periodontal abscess. The clinician should also be concerned regarding the possible loss of positional stability of the abutment tooth, potentially leading to over-eruption of this or the opposing tooth, with the following consequences of having to re-prepare the abutment and to take a new impression.

## Fractured and loose temporary crowns

Management of the loose temporary crown includes an immediate recementation or replacement. Following three factors should be considered:

(1) *Strength of the temporary crown*: Is the material strong enough? Is the preparation adequate and does it allow sufficient thickness to the temporary crowns?
(2) *Strength of the cement*: A strong alternative cement should be considered in the case of a non-retentive preparation.

(3) *Occlusal forces:* These are also a major factor in the repeated loss of temporary crowns. Therefore, a thorough occlusal examination is of paramount importance. This should include the static and functional occlusion as well as the possible presence of parafunctional habits, such as clenching or bruxism.

A repeatedly failing temporary crown could be indicative of underpreparation or heavy occlusal forces, and could be a predictor of a future failing permanent crown if these problems are not addressed.

## Fractured and loose permanent crowns and bridges

Mobility of a permanent crown (retainer in the case of a bridge) could be caused by a number of things. Box 5.2 provides the practitioner with a checklist for the most likely reasons.

---

**Box 5.2   Most likely reasons for loose permanent crowns and bridges**

(1) *Crown decementation, which in turn could be due to:*
   a. non-retentive preparation;
   b. secondary caries;
   c. weak (or dissolved) cement (or loosening of the crown retention screw on an implant);
   d. excessive occlusal forces.
(2) *Crown fracture*
   This can be seen with porcelain but not metal crowns. It could be due to:
   a. insufficient porcelain thickness as a result of tooth underpreparation;
   b. excessive occlusal forces.
(3) *Abutment fracture, because of:*
   a. secondary caries;
   b. excessive occlusal forces.
(4) *Fracture/decementation of a post or loosening of the abutment screw on an implant as a result of:*
   a. dissolved cement/secondary caries;
   b. use of weak post;
   c. excessive occlusal forces.

---

### Single crowns

The literature shows a wide variance between figures on failure rates. This is due to the myriad of differences in clinical techniques, occlusal characteristics, laboratory techniques and criteria for repair or replacement.

Management includes cleaning all cement residues off the abutment to carefully inspect for any caries or fractures. If both the abutment and crown are deemed sound and usable, the crown should be cleaned of all cement and its fit checked. This includes an inspection of the margin's relation to the preparation and gingivae as well as the contact points. Before the crown is recemented, it is very important that occlusion is checked both in ICP and in lateral and protrusive excursions. Certain crowns will also require treatment of the fitting surface before recementation, including sand-blasting and acid-etching.

A variety of permanent cements are at the clinician's disposal. While it is not the scope of this book to discuss the choice of cement, it should be remembered that a stronger cement to that used originally might be indicated, such as resin cements, especially in cases of non-retentive abutments or heavy occlusal forces. However, this does not eliminate the need for a careful check of the crown design and the applied occlusal forces, which with the use a stronger cement might affect the stability of the abutment as opposed the crown.

If the crown is deemed unusable in the longer term, the abutment should be temporarily protected by either a new temporary crown or the same old crown cemented with a temporary cement. In the former case, the dentist will often find it helpful to take an alginate impression with the old crown in situ to use it as a matrix for the chairside temporary crown.

Should the underlying structure (abutment/post) be found deficient due to caries or fracture, that problem needs to be addressed first. On the basis of its severity and extension, a decision is made whether it is possible to recement the dislodged crown in the same visit. The clinician may also wish to use the crown as a matrix to build the broken down abutment. This technique is described in texts on restorative dentistry.

However, in many cases, an immediate reconstruction of the abutment may be deemed inappropriate and a new treatment plan needed including root canal treatment, restoration of the abutment core, replacement of the fractured post, or even extraction of the abutment tooth.

## Bridges

Failure rates are considerably higher in bridges than in single crowns. Clinicians should beware of radiopaque crowns and bridges 'hiding' caries radiographically.

Management of failing bridges is different to that for single crowns in that when the bridge debonds from one side, the clinician faces the dilemma of having to remove the intact cemented retainer. Excessive forces during attempted removal of the bridge may irreversibly damage the abutment. Alternative options include the following:

• Sectioning the intact cemented retainer and making a new fixed bridge.
• Sectioning the bridge between the pontic and loose retainer, and leaving the remaining units as a cantilever bridge. The loose retainer will be then recemented or remade.

- Attempting to recement the loose retainer. This technique has been recently described but not followed-up in the long term. The method comprises making a hole in the loose retainer to inject a resin cement.

Bridge fractures are often caused by breakage in the connector between the pontic and the retainer. Should this happen, the clinician needs to decide whether the broken bridge can be used as it comprises of a separate cantilever bridge one side and a retainer on the other. Alternatively, the two sections could be removed and soldered, or the bridge remade. Other methods have been described to join the two segments in the mouth, but these techniques have not been examined in terms of long-term results.

Whatever the choice, careful examination of the bridge design, the span length and occlusal forces is vital to avoid further failure or additional complications.

## Fracture of the porcelain veneer of a porcelain-fused-to-metal crown

An urgent request to repair a chipped or fractured porcelain veneer for a PFM crown is commonly seen. Different things could cause such veneers to fracture including impact trauma and occlusal forces either excessive or normal on a bridge that has been badly designed (long span).

Immediate management includes a chairside repair of the fractured veneer with composite. The alternative option to remove the crown or bridge in order to fix them in the laboratory or for replacement could prove very difficult, costly and risky to the abutment tooth. This is in addition to the aesthetic challenge until the prosthesis comes back from the laboratory.

Bonding composite to exposed metal involves primarily achieving macro-mechanical retention by making grooves and notches or by abrading the surface. Bonding to exposed porcelain involves abrading, hydrofluoric acid etching and silanating, followed by conventional bonding procedures. Composite patching remains however, a temporary solution as composite repairs are not predictable in terms of longevity, and not as colour stable as porcelain.

Regardless of the chosen method, a careful examination of the bridge design and applied occlusal forces remains essential in avoiding future incidence.

## Fractured and loose posts (dowels)

As previously noted, mobility of a crown or a retainer could be due to mobility of the underlying core and post. This in turn could be caused by loss of retention or fracture in the post. However, root fractures and periodontal complications have also been frequently recorded.

Dental posts are available in numerous types and designs including custom cast posts, prefabricated serrated parallel-sided metal posts, fibre posts and more recently porcelain posts. The first two types are most commonly used. Therefore, it is not surprising to note different survival rates and causes for failure among the various post types. In general, mean survival time for all types have been recorded as 7–11 years. Tapered posts are associated with a higher risk of tooth fracture than are parallel-sided posts. On the other hand, prefabricated metal posts show more post fractures and less frequent root fractures than tapered posts.

Patients with loose or fractured posts may present complaining of tooth mobility with or without pain and/or discomfort. A thorough examination is essential to make a differential diagnosis and achieve the best management. The examination should follow the same rules and guides as described for any other mobility, including palpation and manipulation of the mobile tooth part, and the elimination of possibility of a root fracture or periodontal abscess. Radiographs will often be helpful; however, they should be interpreted carefully as the fracture line in the root or post could be indistinguishable.

Immediate management should aim to remove the mobile prosthesis and attempt to temporise the abutment tooth. However, the decision-making depends on a number of factors including the following:

- Type and severity of the underlying problem, e.g. tooth fracture vs. loose post.
- Position of the tooth in the mouth, i.e. the aesthetic and functional implications of removing the crown with or without immediate replacement.
- The post material.

Given the possibility that re-inserting the post in place after it has been removed for investigation might be impossible, it is highly recommended that the clinician takes an alginate impression before attempting to remove the crown and underlying post in order to make a temporary post and crown. This is particularly important if the tooth is in the aesthetic zone.

Having completed the examination, the clinician will be faced with a number of possibilities depending on the aforementioned factors.

Starting from the simplest situation, if the post is decemented, but both the tooth and the post or crown complex are judged to be sound, management involves recementation of the post. Nonetheless, it is crucial that the clinician checks occlusal forces to exclude any overload possibility and to avoid the risk of more severe complications in the future, for example, tooth fracture.

If the post is fractured, but the tooth is deemed sound and restorable, the post has to be removed and replaced later with a new one. This procedure might be time consuming as part of the fractured post will be locked inside the root canal. *It also comes with risks of tooth fracture and perforation and is best performed by a restorative specialist.* A judgement needs to be made whether the remaining part should be removed immediately to allow the making of a new temporary post and crown for aesthetic reasons, or whether a temporary 'capping' of the tooth is sufficient to prevent further contamination of the root canal with saliva and food trapping. Removal of the fractured post will largely depend on its type and material as well as the tooth position in the mouth with the associated difficulty in accessing the tooth. The removal could be completed in a number of ways, including the following:

- Holding the broken fragment with fine forceps and turning it anticlockwise.
- Breaking the cement and dislodging the fragment using the ultrasonic tips.
- The Masserann technique.

The Masserann technique, best performed by a specialist, involves the use of hollow tubes specially designed for the removal of intra-canal metallic objects. These tubes (drills) can be operated manually using a screwdriver-like device or mounted on the slow handpiece. Either way, the head of the tube engages the locked instrument and drills a channel in the sound dentine around it. The procedure continues until the post fragment becomes loose in place, and can be then forced out using a small spoon excavator or a probe. Once this is removed, a prefabricated metal or fibre post can be used to support a composite temporary crown made using the impression previously taken. If upon examination the tooth is found fractured and is beyond restoration, it is sensible to extract the tooth and make a temporary bridge, if this is required and achievable.

## Fractured and loose implants

Despite the relatively very high success rate of implants (between 85% and 95%), it is not uncommon for the practitioner to receive a request for emergency management of a failing implant or one of its components. In most cases, it is highly recommended to refer the patient to the specialist who provided the implant; however, this may not be always possible.

Early failure of implants is not commonly encountered in the dental emergency clinic, as patients are usually advised to seek immediate specialist care, if needed. However, late implant failure is likely to be encountered in the first place by the general dental practitioner or presentation to a practitioner working in DEC. Late failures are usually associated with moderate to severe bone loss, mostly located in posterior areas, and involve a multi-unit prosthesis. When presenting as an emergency, patients usually worry of the implant mobility as well as the inflammation in surrounding tissues. Management of the latter has been discussed previously.

When the clinician is faced with a mobile implant, a full examination of the implant and its parts should be undertaken. Mobility could be caused at different levels as follows:

- *At the fixture level*: This is a case of failing osseointegration and similar to loss of periodontal/bone support. Another reason could be a fracture of the fixture (which is less likely).
- *At the abutment level*: Abutment could become loose if the abutment screw is loosened.
- *At the crown level*: The crown could become loose if it decements or the retention screw becomes loose.

The aforementioned describes a single tooth implant. However, it is not possible to cover the various possibilities of failure for all types of implant-retained fixed or removable prostheses within the scope of this book. A careful management approach will be required for each case separately, including manipulation of the mobile component, radiographs and occlusal examination.

The practitioner is reminded that management of implant-related problems should always be reversible and minimal as much as possible.

## Fractures and swallowing of removable prostheses

### Denture fracture

Although a broken denture is not usually perceived by the dentist as a major concern, this may have significant implications on the patient's everyday life.

Fracture may involve any part of the denture. Any solution to repair the denture remains less ideal to making a new one. The ratio of fracture of upper to lower denture is 1:3. The most common reason for fracture is accidental dropping of the denture in case of the lower and improper fit and stability of the denture and improper arrangement and occlusion of the teeth for the upper.

### Immediate management

The clinician needs to make a judgement of the urgency and type of the repair needed. Chairside repair might be indicated to repair the acrylic parts (acrylic base and tooth) in urgent cases. Cases involving metal parts of the denture will require repair by soldering the broken part or making a new clasp.

### Denture swallowing

Swallowing or aspiration of a removable partial denture occurs more frequently in the elderly or psychiatrically ill population, and represents a serious medical situation. The complications arising from swallowed removable prostheses include, but are not limited to, laceration, perforation, and haemorrhage of the oesophagus and gastrointestinal tract. These in turn could cause peritonitis, septicaemia, or result in foreign body granulomas and abscess formation.

### Other problems

Other denture-related problems have been reported earlier in this chapter (see Section 'Stomatitis').

It is not within the scope of this book to cover other denture-related problems such as over-extended or under-extended dentures, non-retentive dentures and so forth.

## Conclusions

Dental emergencies are often of a restorative nature. It is important that any clinician working in a dental emergency clinic is acquainted with the basics of management.

It is essential that the clinician is able to quickly establish the correct diagnosis and effective treatment for the clinical problem. The key to successful diagnosis and management can be summarised in the following three areas:

(1) Good history taking, thorough examination and special tests where indicated.
(2) Control of pain and/or infection.
(3) Emergency treatment planning that will not mitigate against a definitive treatment plan.

This chapter has not attempted to cover every possible emergency scenario of a restorative nature that could be encountered, but has illustrated some of the more common presentations and differential diagnoses.

## Further reading

Roger-Leroi V, Lalechere-Lestradfe C, Tubert-Jeannin S (2007) Characteristics of the patients needing emergency dental treatment at the hospital of Clermont-Ferrand (France). *Rev Epidemiol Sante Publique* **55**(3), 197–202.

Scully C (1995) The pattern of patient attendance for emergency care in a British dental teaching hospital. *Community Dental Health* **12**(3), 151–154.

# Chapter 6

# Acute Presentations of Chronic Oro-Facial Pain Conditions

**J. Durham**

## Introduction

Pain is a highly subjective experience and has been defined as occurring when and where the patient says it does. Pain is defined by the International Association for the Study of Pain as 'an unpleasant sensory and emotional experience associated with actual or potential tissue damage, or described in terms of such damage'. It is difficult to determine a cut-off point for when acute becomes chronic pain but estimates vary from 3 to 12 months. Chronic pain conditions affecting the oro-facial region can originate from any of the multitude of tissue types present in the head and neck: vascular, nervous, muscular, bony and cartilage, amongst others.

Chronic pain conditions must start at a chronological point. They can start either insidiously, or suddenly with an acute limitation of everyday function due to the severity and urgency of the pain experienced. In the latter case, patients may present 'acutely' to the dental practitioner. The presentation of their complaint may be complicated by the rich sensory oro-facial peripheral innervations. Messages from the peripheral nociceptors can diverge or converge, and therefore, pain may be reported, felt and perceived, to be related to teeth or other oral structures, but may originate from another anatomical site.

The aim of this chapter is to outline the characteristics and *initial* management of the more common chronic oro-facial pain conditions that might present acutely to a dental emergency clinic. It is not intended to be a complete manual for the management of chronic oro-facial pain. Suggestions for further reading in the field and supportive references for the text are given at the end of the chapter.

*Dental Emergencies*, First Edition. Edited by Mark Greenwood and Ian Corbett.
© 2012 Blackwell Publishing Ltd. Published 2012 by Blackwell Publishing Ltd.

## Oro-facial pain history

Patients may describe oro-facial pain using a rich variety of terms but unfortunately the terms chosen do not always distinguish between the differing origins of the pain. What will nearly always be communicated is the particularly high intensity of oro-facial pain. The aim of this section is to give an overview of a brief oro-facial pain history and highlight some of the symptoms and characteristics of the commonly presenting chronic oro-facial pain conditions. Throughout the section it is important to bear in mind that as pain is subjective these classical descriptors, or signs, are not true in every case.

There are two issues of overriding importance to consider when taking an oro-facial pain history. The first is to ensure that the practitioner establishes a degree of empathy with the patient with regard to their complaint. The second is to establish that their complaint has legitimacy and ensure an attempt is made to provide a diagnosis, even if provisional, by the end of the consultation. A good, empathic oro-facial pain history and provisional diagnosis may have almost therapeutic effects on the level of stress and anxiety patients with oro-facial pain will experience, often due to a long and complex journey through the health service.

The history-taking format follows that described in Chapter 2. That is, to begin with the chief or presenting complaint, proceeding through the history of the presenting complaint, medical history, social history, dental history and then move onto examining the patient, remembering of course that the examination actually starts when the patient first enters the room.

Patients with oro-facial pain may report two or more interlinked chief complaints but describe them as a single complaint. If it is felt that this is the case, it is important to discuss this with the patient and clarify whether or not there are two or more definite, separate, issues/diagnoses, or that they are indeed one complaint. This will help to make taking the history of the presenting complaint easier and create less confusion in the clinician and patients' minds. It may also make diagnosis and treatment easier. If there are indeed multiple complaints, this should be made clear in the notes by enumerating the complaints so that anyone reading the notes can quickly reference and relate findings and diagnoses to complaints.

In the history of the presenting complaint, the practitioner should specifically examine the characteristics of the pain(s) (see also Chapter 2) and as a minimum enquire about the following:

- *Location, radiation and referral*: Ask the patient to take *one* finger and point to where the pain starts, then ask them to show with that *single* finger where it radiates or refers to.
- *Onset and duration*: Specifically, how frequently is the pain occurring, or is it constant? If it is constant, are there acute exacerbations against a background of constant pain?
- *Quality of pain*. Ask the patient to describe the type of pain they are experiencing, e.g. stabbing, burning, aching, etc.

- *Magnitude*: Ask on a scale of 1–10, 10 being the worst imaginable pain, firstly where would they rank their pain generally, and secondly where would they rank it today?
- *Relieving and precipitating factors.*
- *Diurnal and seasonal variation.*
- *Brief sleep history*:
  - Do they sleep well or do they wake excessively early?
  - Does the pain wake them from sleep?
  - Does the pain stop them getting to sleep?
  - Is the pain worse when they wake up?
- *Effects of the pain on their everyday lives*: Gently and tactfully attempt to gain an understanding of the impact the pain is having on the patient's everyday life, e.g. their job, close relationships etc. This is important, as patients with oro-facial pain can need social support with their everyday lives until the pain is controlled. Without appropriate social support from their closest family and friends, the pain may worsen in certain conditions due to increased stress and anxiety.
- *Surgical therapy prior to the pain*: Recent dental, medical and surgical therapy *prior* to this pain.
- *Previous experience*: Experience of this type of pain and previous treatment for it. Within this, ask the patient to list the treatments in chronological order and detail how effective they found the treatment. It is also useful to note the doses of medications they have tried previously and any side effects. Some patients may find this very difficult, and if this is the case, their family doctor or dentist should be consulted for further details.
- *Systemic symptoms*: When pain occurs, e.g. lacrimation, rhinorrhoea, dizziness, palpitations, weakness, nausea, vomiting, photo- or phonophobia.
- *Systemic well-being*: Recent weight loss, lymphadenopathy elsewhere in the body, sensory or motor deficits elsewhere, pain elsewhere in body.

If the pain history is somewhat unclear, then the use of a pain diary by the patient over a week or two might help clarify matters. This diary can be as simple or as complex as the clinician desires, some good examples can be found in the literature. It may be best to refer the patient at this stage to a specialist clinic so that the pain diary can be reviewed.

Characteristics of pain from different tissue types do differ slightly, but as one would expect there can be a large amount of crossover. To further complicate things, it is also possible to have two types of pain occurring simultaneously, or to have one type of pain exacerbating another type of pain for example, acute pulpitis exacerbating a temporomandibular disorder. Table 6.1 gives a summary of the characteristics of pain occurring from different tissue types in the oro-facial region, but as explained in the preceding sentence it is a guide rather than absolute.

The medical history should be taken as described previously in Chapter 2, with special attention given to anything discovered in the enquiries made in the history of presenting complaint. The social history is as standard, but it

**Table 6.1** Characteristics of chronic oro-facial pain.

| | Pain of odontogenic origin | Pain of neurovascular origin | Pain of musculoskeletal origin | Neuropathic pain |
|---|---|---|---|---|
| Localisation | Usually, well localised to a particular tooth | Not necessarily well localised, may be bilateral or unilateral | Not necessarily well localised, may be bilateral or unilateral Often overlies in broad areas the musculoskeletal structure causing the pain Pain radiates and refers frequently, including to teeth | Can be well localised to a dermatome if trigeminal neuralgia or to area of trauma, e.g. previous extraction site if traumatic neuropathy |
| Character | Sharp, high intensity and constant type of pain | Throbbing, vascular quality Stabbing or boring Transient, periodic pain of varying duration. Usually associated autonomic signs, e.g. lacrimation (tearing) | Aching type of pain Constant with acute exacerbations linked to increased stress or function | Paroxysmal sharp, electrical stabbing, needle-like pain if neuralgia If traumatic neuropathy, can be burning aching, or 'itchy' |
| Sleep | If irreversible, pulpitis can wake patient from sleep | Can wake patient from sleep | If nocturnal parafunction involved, pain can be worse after sleep, if daytime parafunction, it can be worse before sleep | |

**Table 6.1** (Continued).

| | Pain of odontogenic origin | Pain of neurovascular origin | Pain of musculoskeletal origin | Neuropathic pain |
|---|---|---|---|---|
| Local provocation | Exacerbates with hot, cold | Photo or Phonophobia Nausea and/or vomiting | Palpation of structure involved usually provokes pain Dynamic testing of musculo-skeletal system area suspected of being cause of pain usually produces pain | Palpation of area affected can start pain |
| Allodynia and hyper-algesia | Tooth sometimes tender to bite onto Hyperalgesia to hot and cold | Infrequent allodynia | Allodynia of muscles and joints involved | Allodynia Can even be to normal movement in the case of trigeminal neuralgia |

may be possible at this stage to try and build an understanding of the work-life stressors and events the patient may be experiencing that may be contributory to the pain. The dental history for a patient with oro-facial pain should focus on any treatments that occurred *prior* to the pain, and any treatments *performed for* the pain.

## Examination of patients with oro-facial pain

The examination should be conducted extra-orally and intra-orally as described in Chapter 2. Of specific importance in the extra-oral examination of a patient with oro-facial pain are:

- General appearance and demeanour.
- Any facial grimaces, or tics associated with pain.
- Palpation of the masticatory musculature. All muscles should be thoroughly palpated from insertion to origin to see if this palpation reproduces the patient's pain. If the patient reports any tenderness or restriction in the neck, consideration should also be given to palpating the sternocleidomastoid muscle, posterior intrinsic muscles of the neck and trapezius.
- Palpation (auscultation) and observation of the range of movement of temporomandibular joint (TMJ), specifically examining for clicks, crepitus, deviation or restricted translation of the joint.

- Measurement of the range of movement of the TMJ (parentheses indicate normal values range):
  - Protrusive (6–8 mm)
  - Excursive (6–8 mm)
  - Opening (40–50 mm)
- Palpation of temporal arteries.
- Lymph node examination.
- Salivary gland examination via palpation (bimanual for submandibular).
- Palpation of maxillary air sinuses extra-orally.
- Cranial nerve examination. Disturbances in cranial nerve function should always be taken seriously and fully investigated by an appropriate specialist. (See Chapter 2).
- Auriscopy (otoscopy) can be carried out if competent to do so. If not competent simply, visually inspect the auricle and the visible part of the external auditory meatus and make arrangements for someone competent to conduct an aural examination, if necessary.
- Consideration can be given to a neurological examination if competent to do so and signs and symptoms dictate.

Of specific importance in the intra-oral examination of the patient are:

- Provocation testing of any dental structures implicated by the patient's history, e.g. palpation of ridge, percussion, or Tooth sleuth® testing of teeth.
- Thorough mucosal screening including visualisation of the oropharynx.
- Examine the patient's occlusion. Specifically examine for gross occlusal discrepancies, e.g. a crown high in the occlusion or an overerupted tooth. If competent to do so and if it is indicated conduct a full occlusal examination including noting shim stock contacts, excursive guidance, and non-working side/working side interferences.

## Red flag signs and symptoms

Patients and clinicians are justifiably concerned when acute oro-facial pain presents. Pain can often mean damage or disease. This is not always true, but there are a number of 'red flag' signs and symptoms associated with pain presenting oro-facially that every clinician should be aware of and take prompt action over, either by instituting expedient investigation and treatment, or seeking an urgent specialist opinion. These red flags are included in Table 6.2.

Again, it must be remembered that these 'red flags' are not absolute. They are, however, useful to guide clinicians and if present they should be investigated and an explanation sought for them.

## Special investigations for oro-facial pain

A thorough history and clinical examination will often give sufficient information to make a (clinical) diagnosis in oro-facial pain. Occasionally, the clinician

**Table 6.2** Red flag signs and symptoms.

| | |
|---|---|
| Headache | Worrisome characteristics (SSNOOP – American Headache Society): |
| | **S**ystemic disease or symptoms, e.g. weight loss/gain, malaise, lymphadenopathy<br>**S**econdary headache risk factors, e.g. previous history of malignancy<br>**N**eurological signs or symptoms, e.g. unexplained weakness or cranial nerve dysfunction<br>**O**nset abrupt – 'thunderclap'<br>**O**lder (>50 yr) and new onset headache<br>**P**revious headache history or progression. First ever headache of huge severity or very sudden progression to this level |
| | Specific features of headache:<br>• Precipitated by cough, sneeze or straining<br>• Rousing patient from sleep<br>• On standing<br>• On lying down |
| Ear and nose and throat signs or symptoms | Recurrent epistaxis<br>Anosmia<br>Persistent nasal obstruction or purulent discharge<br>*Objective* hearing loss<br>Lymphadenopathy |
| Oral and maxillofacial signs and symptoms | Near absolute trismus precluding careful oral examination<br>Erythroplakia, erythroleukoplakia, leukoplakia or frank ulceration of oral mucosa<br>Cranial nerve dysfunction especially in cranial nerves five or seven<br>Previous head and neck carcinoma<br>Pre-auricular masses<br>Young onset (<40 yr) trigeminal neuralgia, especially females |

will need to perform specific imaging to help exclude pathology. Dependent on the clinical presentation such imaging may include the following:

• *Plain radiographs*: As indicated and justified by the history and examination.
• *Cone beam computed tomography of teeth*: To examine features of teeth, or pathology associated with them that plain dental radiography cannot identify.
• *Computed tomography of the head and neck*: To exclude head and neck malignancy mimicking an oro-facial pain condition, e.g. sudden onset near absolute trismus of unknown cause in an elderly patient.

- *Magnetic resonance imaging (MRI) of the head*: To exclude vascular compression of the trigeminal nerve root, multiple sclerosis, or intra-cranial pathology such as tumours at the cerbellopontine angle.

It is inadvisable to perform investigations simply because of a request from a patient, especially if there is no clinical indication to do so. These types of requests should be explored with the patient, as if they are worried over a potential sinister cause and there is no clinical objective evidence of such a pathology; extensive reassurance and explanation of the symptoms should be given. If these requests are not explored and explanation and reassurance are not given, the situation is likely to be self-perpetuating and may help worsen the pain experienced.

Haematological investigations may or may not be necessary for patients with oro-facial pain depending on the presentation. Most often, haematological investigations will be undertaken to establish a baseline before commencing pharmacological therapy that may potentially alter aspects of the patient's physiology. However, some oro-facial pain conditions do require haematological investigations to help confirm the clinical diagnosis, for example temporal arteritis, or to exclude an underlying problem, for example burning mouth syndrome.

## Presentation, investigations and initial management of acute non-odontogenic oro-facial pain

This section will *briefly* outline the presenting features of the more common acute presentations of non-odontogenic oro-facial pain by their origin grouping. This section is not an exhaustive text on the various types of chronic oro-facial pain but aims to cover those more likely to present acutely to the dental practitioner.

### Pain of musculoskeletal origin

#### Temporal arteritis

Temporal arteritis can present acutely in the above 50 years age group. There is no gender predilection. Temporal arteritis should be suspected if the following signs and symptoms present:

- Headache in the temporal region.
- Older (>50 years of age) age group.
- Visual disturbances.
- Claudication when eating. Patients can complain of tiredness in moving the jaw when eating.
- Palpably tender and inflamed superficial arteries.

This condition is commonly managed by rheumatologists, but can present in dental clinics. Urgent referral to a rheumatologist is necessary and investigations conducted should include an erythrocyte sedimentation rate and C-reactive protein (CRP) level (see Appendix 1), both of which would be markedly raised, and an urgent temporal artery biopsy. Treatment is by high-dose systemic steroids. If there is a high index of clinical suspicion, treatment should not be delayed by the results of the temporal artery biopsy, as temporal arteritis can cause significant ophthalmological ischaemic complications leading to blindness.

## Musculoskeletal conditions causing painful limited opening

The descriptive term used for the sign and symptoms of limited opening is trismus. Trismus has a diverse aetiology (Table 6.3) and is not itself pathognomic of any particular cause. The specific clinical features of the trismus, in association with other associated signs and symptoms can, however, lead to a diagnosis of the cause of the trismus. Table 6.3 outlines some of the more common acute causes of trismus and the Section 'Myofascial pain with limited mouth opening' discusses some of the chronic oro-facial pain conditions that present with a painful and limited opening. When making a purely clinical diagnosis of one of the chronic oro-facial pain conditions as the cause of trismus, the clinician *must be certain* that they have *excluded any other pathological cause*, such as those listed in Table 6.3, and they must also be prepared to reconsider their diagnosis if the patient does not respond to treatment as expected.

### Myofascial pain with limited mouth opening

This temporomandibular disorder can present acutely. Temporomandibular disorders generally occur between the second and fourth decades and despite occurring equally in both genders, females tend to present more

**Table 6.3**  Other causes of acute trismus.

| Origin | Potential cause |
|---|---|
| Infective | Pericoronitis<br>Collections of pus in tissue spaces (particularly submasseteric space) |
| Neoplastic | Oropharyngeal malignancy |
| Traumatic | Fractures of mandible (particularly condyle, coronoid or ramus)<br>Depressed fracture of zygoma (especially arch fractures)<br>Mucosal trauma from buccally placed upper molar teeth (particularly third molars) |
| Inflammatory | Post-surgery or dental treatment<br>Post-inferior dental nerve block |

frequently than males. Myofascial pain with limited opening may be more prevalent around stressful life events, for example forthcoming examinations and so forth. The patient generally presents with a sudden onset of limited opening with pain around the major jaw closing musculature.

A diagnosis of myofascial pain with limited opening can be made if three or more masticatory muscular sites are tender, pain-free unassisted opening is less than 40 mm and assisted opening achieves 5 mm or more opening than unassisted mouth opening. The ability to greatly assist the mouth opening is in direct contrast to another temporomandibular disorder that causes limited opening due to mechanical dysfunction, disc displacement without reduction with limited opening (see later section).

There is no evidence-based gold standard management for myofascial pain. What is indicated though, is a conservative and reversible approach to management. Initial management of the acute presentation may include a short (less than 2 weeks) course of low-dose benzodiazepines, an intra-oral appliance (such as a lower soft splint), moist heat applied to the musculature affected, non-steroidal anti-inflammatory drugs (NSAIDs), and simple stretching exercises. Stretching can be facilitated by the judicious use of spatulas as shown in (Figure 6.1).

Other options include 'spray and stretch', trigger point injection, acupuncture, physiotherapy and more advanced intra-oral appliances. What is paramount is ensuring the patient is reviewed, as once therapy is instituted the limited opening should start to resolve and if it does not, or it worsens, the diagnosis should be reconsidered and specialist advice or referral sought immediately.

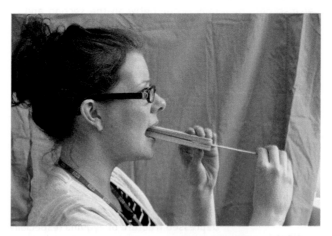

**Figure 6.1** The use of spatulas in encouraging increased mouth opening in cases of trismus. Gently inserting further spatulas as shown can lead to improved mouth opening by gentle stretching. (From Moore, U.J. (ed.) (2011) *Principles of Oral and Maxillofacial Surgery*, 6th edn. Oxford: Wiley-Blackwell. With permission from John Wiley & Sons Ltd.)

## Disc displacement without reduction and with limited opening (DDwoRLO)

As DDwoRLO is a temporomandibular disorder, its age group and gender predilection mirrors that of myofascial pain with limited opening. The patient generally presents with a sudden limitation in mouth opening with pain affecting the TMJ(s) occurring in the last few days. A careful history is needed to help make the diagnosis of DDwoRLO as the clinician needs to ascertain whether or not the patient has been aware of a click in their TMJ previously and which side this was attributed to. If there was a click, this was on the side that is now more painful, and this disappeared with the acute limitation in opening, the diagnosis may be all but made. Full examination should include excluding other potential causes of trismus as detailed for myofascial pain with limited opening. In contrast to myofascial pain with limited opening, the clinician will not significantly be able to assist opening due to the mechanical 'blocking' effect of the displaced disc.

The diagnosis of DDwoRLO can be made clinically if on examination the patient exhibits: less than 35 mm of painful mouth opening; less than 5 mm of passive stretch on assisted opening that is painful on the affected joint and less than 7 mm of contralateral excursion or uncorrected deviation towards the affected side. MRI of the affected joint can be requested if the clinician desires, but this is not absolutely necessary in the acute phase and initial management can begin without the imaging if a clinical diagnosis can be made with confidence.

Initial management of DDwoRLO should always be conservative and reversible as evidence suggests that this type of management achieves similar results to more invasive therapy. Schiffman et al in 2007, demonstrated that there was no difference between surgical approaches to DDwoRLO and medical management/rehabilitation. If Schiffman et al's approach is adopted, medical management and rehabilitation of this acute disorder would involve the following:

- *A muscle relaxant at night-time*: The author's preference is to consider a short course of Diazepam subject to no contraindications.
- *Anti-inflammatory medication*: Dependent on patient preference Schiffman et al instituted a 6-day reducing dose of systemic prednisolone, or high-dose Ibuprofen. If systemic steroids were employed, high-dose ibuprofen was started on the seventh day of treatment. The author's decision on the utilisation of steroids is dependent on contraindications and level of discomfort the patient reports. If the reported level of discomfort is low, the author institutes NSAIDs alone subject to no contraindications.
- *Physiotherapy:* A wide range of physiotherapeutic modalities were employed by Schiffman et al.
- *Intra-oral appliance*: From the description given in Schiffman et al's paper, a stabilisation splint was employed. It is sometimes difficult to provide such a splint with restricted mouth opening and a lower soft splint may be an adequate substitute whilst mouth opening improves.

- *Cognitive behavioural therapy*: This may not be readily accessible in every unit but can often be arranged via the patient's general medical practitioner.
- *Moist heat or ice and dietary changes*: Self-applied moist heat or ice and conservative advice on temporary dietary changes, and habit modification.

Other options for managing this disorder in the acute phase include an arthrocentesis or arthroscopy to try and displace the disc back to its near normal position in relation to the condylar head.

A more conservative option that is less evidence-based is to attempt a self, or manual, reduction of the disc within the first week of the displacement. Patients can attempt to self reduce the disc displacement by consciously attempting to relax their masticatory musculature and then perform a maximal lateral excursion away from the affected joint. Once they have achieved this maximal lateral excursion, they should then attempt to open whilst maintaining their lateral position. The premise is that the maximal lateral excursion will provide as much room in the joint complex as possible for the disc to slip back towards its original position. A manual reduction has been described. Figure 6.2 demonstrates this manual reduction technique, which may require the use of local anaesthesia to the TMJ (Figure 6.3) to aid compliance.

Clinicians beginning the initial acute management of this condition should bear in mind that the vast majority of patients will increase their mouth opening with no more interventions than are necessary to alleviate their discomfort. There is, however, a need for careful specialist review for the similar reason as myofascial pain with limited opening needs review. This is especially true for DDwoRLO as the majority of patients can take up to 18 months of palliative therapy to achieve near maximal mouth opening. The diagnosis must

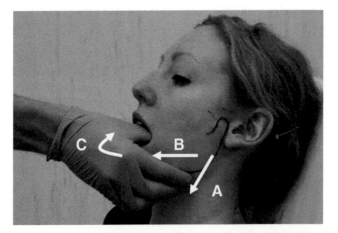

**Figure 6.2** Attempting to manually reduce a non-reduced displaced articular disc. Hand position on the near side (affected side). Gentle distraction force through thumbs and fingers is applied in direction A for a few seconds. Continue the distractive forces and slowly move through direction B towards protrusion and then out into lateral excursion direction C away from the affected side.

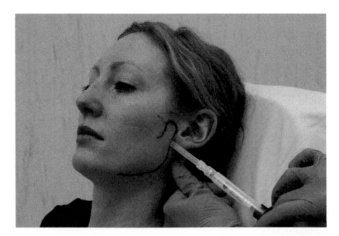

**Figure 6.3** Auriculotemporal nerve block as described by Donlon in 1984. Needle is sheathed for model's safety. Clean the skin with a Steret® and insert needle just below the junction of tragus and ear lobe continuing in an anterosuperior direction until the posterior aspect of the condylar neck is encountered. Once bone is contacted, reorientate needle to manoeuvre it so it is medial to the condyle advance a few more millimetres and *aspirate* prior to injection.

therefore be made with some confidence ensuring no sinister or serious pathology is missed.

## Myospasm of muscles of mastication

Myospasm, 'an acute sudden involuntary, tonic contraction of a muscle' is rare in the masticatory system. It requires an electromyogram (EMG) to definitively confirm its diagnosis. Depending on which muscle of mastication the myospasm affects, it may cause an acute malocclusion, generally some form of open bite. Irrespective of which muscle it affects, it will cause pain and a decreased range of motion. Not all units have the facilities for EMG and if the aim is to clinically manage the patient, a clinical diagnosis by exclusion is reasonable, but careful follow-up should be arranged and the clinician should have a high index of suspicion for other causative pathology. The management of myospasm broadly mirrors that outlined for myofascial pain with limited opening.

### Temporomandibular joint dislocation

This can affect any gender across a wide spectrum of ages. Some of the reasons for dislocations can include the following: laxity in the TMJ ligaments and capsule; overclosure caused by skeletal pattern or excessively worn dentures; traumatic unsupportive extraction technique, and intubation for a general anaesthetic. The patient will present with pain affecting (both) TMJs, an inability to close the mouth and a history suggestive of some form of over-translation of the TMJ(s). Examination often reveals the condylar head(s) to be palpable anterior to the articular eminence and panoramic tomography can be used to confirm this, although this is not mandatory to make the diagnosis. If the dislocation is unilateral, there is usually deviation of the midline towards the unaffected side.

Dislocation of the TMJ(s) is best managed as soon after the event as possible by someone experienced in the reduction of TMJ dislocations. This is for two reasons. Firstly, if a precipitous reduction is performed, there is less time for muscular co-contraction (protective muscular splinting) of the powerful jaw closing musculature, which will make subsequent attempts more difficult. Secondly, if someone inexperienced has several attempts at reducing the dislocation, this is likely to increase muscle splinting and make subsequent attempts more difficult. If performed early, often, reduction can be achieved without the need for local anaesthesia, sedation or general anaesthesia.

Despite highlighting the need for an experienced operator to reduce an acutely presenting dislocation, it is not unreasonable to attempt reduction once or twice prior to seeking specialist advice, especially if one is located some distance from the nearest specialist centre. One of the simplest methods to attempt reduction of an acute dislocation in a conscious patient is to stimulate their gag reflex by touching either their soft palate or the posterior wall of their oropharynx with the handle of a dental mirror. It is advisable to discuss this with the patient prior to doing so. If this is successful, the reduction can be incredibly quick and powerful, so all fingers should be kept out of the mouth and care should be taken to avoid trauma to the teeth from the handle of the mirror.

The traditional reduction technique is to place the patient in a dental chair with their head well supported. The clinician stands in front of the patient placing their thumbs intra-orally on the lower molar teeth or the external oblique ridge. It is advisable if placing the thumbs on teeth to protect them by either binding with gauze or placing tongue spatulas beneath them.

The clinician should then explain to the patient that all the way through the reduction they should consciously attempt to relax the muscles of their face as the natural inclination is to contract their jaw-closing muscles to counteract the force applied downwards by the clinician. One subtle way of trying to achieve this is to cause inhibition of the jaw-closing musculature by asking the patient to consciously attempt to yawn during the downwards pressure exerted by the clinician through the teeth/external oblique ridge.

The downwards pressure on the posterior teeth/external oblique ridge should be increased gradually through the teeth and if attempting bilateral reduction one side should be concentrated on at a time; indeed, the contralateral side may reduce almost spontaneously once the ipsilateral side reduces. The downward pressure aims to distract the mandible beneath the apex of the articular eminence, and once this is achieved, posterior pressure is added to the downwards pressure in an attempt to slide the condylar head back over the eminence and into the glenoid fossa.

If several unsuccessful attempts are made at reduction, it is advisable to consider a pharmacological adjunct to the reduction. This may be in the form of local anaesthesia of the TMJ, benzodiazepine sedation or general anaesthesia. The non-specialist should not, however, make several attempts at reduction and should seek specialist referral well before the need for pharmacological adjuncts.

### Pain of neurovascular origin

There are several trigeminal autonomic cephalgias that are very rare and are outside the scope of this chapter. Further information on these and other oro-facial pains of neurovascular origin can be found in several excellent texts.

The most common neurovascular pain is migraine, which has several forms. It is beyond the scope of the dental practitioner to be aware of the subtleties of each type of migraine, but what they should be aware of are the characteristics of migraine so that is not confused with any other type of oro-facial pain. These signs and symptoms are:

- Persistent throbbing pain unilaterally for up to 72 hours
- Associated systemic complaints of nausea, vomiting, photo or phonophobia
- Pain aggravated by everyday function
- Aura may or may not be present

Management of migraine is commonly started by the patient's family doctor and may or may not involve a neurologist. Firstly, the clinician tries to identify and eliminate any triggers the patient may be aware of, for example caffeine, chocolate. The pharmacological management of migraine is then conducted by the use of one of two management strategies. One strategy aims to prevent migraines from occurring (prophylactic strategy) through the use of long-term systemic medication – for example beta-blockers – whilst the other method aims to stop a migraine in its early phase (abortive strategy) – for example through the use of triptans either intra-nasally, orally or subcutaneously. The choice between the two management strategies largely depends on the frequency of occurrence of the migraine.

### Pain of neuropathic origin

There are multiple types of neuropathy that can produce pain in the oro-facial region. This section aims to cover trigeminal neuralgia, and one specific peripheral neuropathic pain, traumatic neuropathy, and broadly discuss two central neuropathic pains that may or may not be linked: persistent idiopathic facial pain (atypical facial pain) and atypical odontalgia. The reader is referred to the further reading section at the end of this chapter for details of the other types of neuropathic pain affecting the oro-facial region.

### Trigeminal neuralgia

There are a number of sub-classifications of trigeminal neuralgia (TN) that are beyond the scope of this section, for example pre-TN and atypical neuralgia. The 'Further reading' section at the end of this chapter includes texts that cover these sub-classifications in detail. This section will concentrate on classical (primary, idiopathic or essential) TN and secondary TN.

Classical TN is more prevalent in females and presents between the ages of 50 and 70 years. If TN presents prior to this age range, especially before the age of 30 years, the clinician should be suspicious of secondary TN. Secondary TN is caused by a pathology other than vascular compression of the trigeminal nerve root, including tumours at the cerebellopontine angle or in the posterior cranial fossa, and multiple sclerosis. Classical TN is when either vascular compression of the trigeminal nerve root is demonstrated or when no pathology is demonstrated. Therefore, the investigation of choice for all TN is MRI of the head, which will help demonstrate the presence or absence of pathology and vascular compression.

TN generally presents with a paroxysmal, stabbing, often described as 'electric shock-like' or 'hot needle-like', pain affecting one or more of the trigeminal nerve dermatomes. The lower two trigeminal dermatomes are more frequently affected. A trigger usually elicits the pain and there are multiple possible triggers. Some of the more common triggers are talking, chewing, touch and temperature change. The touch trigger can be as light as gusts of cold air or as definite as digital pressure. After the paroxysmal pain, there is generally a refractory period as the nerve has depolarised and needs to repolarise, this means re-provocation of the trigger does not necessarily trigger the pain again.

A thorough history and examination are mandatory and the examination should include full cranial nerve testing. Investigations should include an MRI scan of the head at some point during the individual's management, and baseline full blood count, urea and electrolytes and liver function tests prior to commencing medical management due to the risks of induction of liver enzymes, hyponatraemia, thrombocytopaenia and leucopaenia.

If a clinical diagnosis of classical TN is made prior to advanced imaging, then evidence-based management of TN suggests starting carbamazepine at 300 mg in divided doses (lower to 100–200 mg in very elderly and infirm patients) increasing the dose by 100 mg every third day to a maximum daily dose of 1600 mg. The total daily dose should be divided over two to three doses. Subject to contraindications, nerve blocks of the causative branch of the trigeminal nerve with long-acting local anaesthetics such as bupivacaine can help provide temporary relief from symptoms.

If a non-specialist starts Carbamazepine, it would be advisable to arrange specialist review of the patient as soon as possible, preferably within the first 2 weeks of initiating treatment. Initial specialist review can be performed by oral and maxillofacial surgery or oral medicine. If MRI shows a vascular compression or other pathology, neurosurgical review is mandatory. A neurosurgical microvascular decompression may be recommended.

## Peripheral and central neuropathies

One of the most commonly occurring peripheral neuropathic pains affecting the oro-facial region is damage to either the inferior alveolar or lingual nerves following some form of surgery, the most common being lower third molar removal and implant placement in the mandible.

Seminal work by Robinson et al (2004) has produced guidelines for the presentation of patients with paraesthesia, anaesthesia and dysaesthesia (painful numbness) following lower third molar extraction. Algorithms for management of such patients have been developed but are beyond the scope of this text. In essence, the earlier that a patient is referred to a specialist oral and maxillofacial surgery department for an opinion on ongoing management, the better. Failing resolution after surgery there is no gold standard medical management of persistent dysaesthesia, but topical anaesthetics, anticonvulsants and tricyclic antidepressants may be of some limited benefit.

Management of peripheral traumatic neuropathy caused by dental implant placement has largely focused on the inferior alveolar nerve. Management of lingual nerve damage caused by dental implant treatment would be largely similar to that for lingual nerve damage induced by the removal of the lower third molar as the mechanisms of injury are likely to be similar (Khawaja and Renton 2009; Kraut and Chahal 2002). Two papers in the literature have attempted to provide a protocol for inferior alveolar nerve injury caused by dental implant placement. Both recommend appropriate imaging and immediate removal of the implant if anaesthesia persists or dysaesthesia occurs after placement. This removal is then to be followed, subject to no contraindications and appropriate gastro-protection, by high-dose Ibuprofen and or a tapering dose of systemic prednisolone. This initial management should be followed by careful monitoring of the neurosensory deficit. Paraesthesia that occurs after implant placement will require careful immediate review, preferably by the clinician who performed the implant placement as they will know how surgery proceeded. Investigation and decisions on how to manage the paraesthesia will need to be made on a case-by-case basis by that clinician or in consultation with that clinician. Persisting dysaesthesia following removal of the implant(s) should follow similar lines as outlined for that following lower third molar removal although this is not based on evidence.

## Atypical odontalgia, persistent idiopathic facial pain
The most frequently occurring central neuropathic pains affecting the oro-facial region are atypical odontalgia and persistent idiopathic facial pain (atypical facial pain). Their diagnosis is often one of exclusion; pain from any other source or cause is ruled out and there may be an identifiable precipitating event usually involving a deafferentation injury, e.g. the removal of pulpal tissue or exodontia. Pain may not follow normal anatomical boundaries and teeth investigated may have no discernible pathology. Any patient presenting with these types of signs and symptoms, with no other discernible objective signs of pathology or oro-facial pain condition should not have irreversible therapy until reviewed by a specialist. Management of these conditions is usually through the use of medications with neuromodulatory capacity, for example tricyclic antidepressants, GABA analogues.

## Further reading

de Leeuw R (2008) Internal derangements of the temporomandibular joint. *Oral Maxillofac Surg Clin North Am* **20**, 159-168, v.

de Leeuw R (2008) *Orofacial Pain: Guidelines for Assessment, Diagnosis, and Management*. Quintessence, Chicago.

Donlon WC, Truta MP, Eversole LR (1984) A modified auriculotemporal nerve block for regional anesthesia of the temporomandibular joint. *J Oral Maxillofac Surg* **42**, 544-545.

Durham J et al (2010) Living with uncertainty: temporomandibular disorders. *J Dent Res* **89**, 827-830.

Epstein JB, Jones CK (1993) Presenting signs and symptoms of nasopharyngeal carcinoma. *Oral Surg Oral Med Oral Pathol* **75**, 32-36.

Greene CS (2010) Managing the care of patients with temporomandibular disorders: a new guideline for care. *J Am Dent Assoc* **141**, 1086-1088.

Hasanain F et al (2009) Adapting the diagnostic definitions of the RDC/TMD to routine clinical practice: a feasibility study. *J Dent* **37**, 955-962.

IASP (2007) International Association for the Study of Pain - Pain Terminology. http://www.iasp-pain.org/AM/Template.cfm?Section=Pain_Definitions &Template=/CM/HTMLDisplay.cfm&ContentID=1728#Pain.

Jorns TP, Zakrzewska JM (2007) Evidence-based approach to the medical management of trigeminal neuralgia. *Br J Neurosurg* **21**, 253-261.

Khawaja N, Renton T (2009) Case studies on implant removal influencing the resolution of inferior alveolar nerve injury. *Br Dent J* **206**, 365-370.

Kraut RA, Chahal O (2002) Management of patients with trigeminal nerve injuries after mandibular implant placement. *J Am Dent Assoc* **133**, 1351-1354.

McCaffery M (1968) *Nursing Practice Theories Related to Cognition, Bodily Pain, and Man-environment Interactions*. UCLA at Los Angeles Students' Store, Los Angeles.

Merskey H, Bogduk N (1994) *Classification of Chronic Pain; Description of Chronic Pain Syndromes and Definitions of Pain Terms*. IASP, Seattle.

Okeson JP (2003) *Management of Temporomandibular Disorders and Occlusion*. Mosby, St. Louis.

Okeson JP (2007) Joint intracapsular disorders: diagnostic and non-surgical management considerations. *Dent Clin North Am* **51**, 85-103, vi.

Robinson PP et al (2004) Current management of damage to the inferior alveolar and lingual nerves as a result of removal of third molars. *Br J Oral Maxillofac Surg* **42**, 285-292.

Sato S et al (1997) The natural course of anterior disc displacement without reduction in the temporomandibular joint: follow-up at 6, 12, and 18 months. *J Oral Maxillofac Surg* **55**, 234-238; discussion 238-239.

Schiffman EL et al (2007) Randomized effectiveness study of four therapeutic strategies for TMJ closed lock. *J Dent Res* **86**, 58-63.

Wright EF (2009) *Manual of Temporomandibular Disorders*. Wiley-Blackwell, Oxford.

Yamaguchi T et al (2006) The advantageous direction of jaw movement for releasing TMJ intermittent lock. *Cranio* **24**, 171-178.

Yamaguchi T et al (2007) Condylar movements of temporomandibular disorder patients with intermittent lock: a pilot study. *Cranio* **25**, 50-56.

# Chapter 7
# Traumatic Injuries to the Teeth and Oral Soft Tissues

## U. Chaudhry and I.C. Mackie

## Assessment of the traumatised patient

### History

A comprehensive history should be taken of the traumatised patient at initial presentation. This should allow the clinician to make the decision whether the injury is suitable to be treated in a primary care setting or should be referred to a hospital/dental hospital.

Refer to a general hospital when there is a history of:

- loss of consciousness;
- vomiting;
- headache;
- amnesia;
- persistent coughing;
- difficulties in focusing the eyes.

Once it has been established that the injury is suitable for management in a primary care setting, the following questions relating to the injury should be asked:

- What is the nature of the injury? (If tooth avulsion, note the extra-alveolar dry time, storage medium and if the tooth was contaminated.)
- How, when (include date and time) and where did the injury occur?
- Are all teeth/broken fragments accounted for?
- Is there any disruption in the occlusion?

*Dental Emergencies*, First Edition. Edited by Mark Greenwood and Ian Corbett.
© 2012 Blackwell Publishing Ltd. Published 2012 by Blackwell Publishing Ltd.

## Medical history

General health (cardiac, respiratory, fits/faints, episodes of hospitalisation, endocrine, any current treatment by general practioner or hospital specialist) including tetanus status.

## Examination

The examination of the patient should begin on entering the surgery. The general state of the patient *and* the specific injuries should be noted. The ABCDE approach (see Chapter 11) should be used to assess the injured patient.

### Extra-oral examination
- *Soft tissues*: Facial asymmetry, swellings, bruises, lacerations, puncture wounds.
- *Hard tissues*: Bony step deformity on palpation, deviation/pain on opening/ closing, temporomandibular joint.
- *Diagram*: Draw a rough diagram noting all aforementioned observations.
- The clinician should only attempt suturing when they feel confident in their abilities to achieve an aesthetic and functional result for superficial extra-oral and intra-oral wounds (once thoroughly débrided and cleaned). Gaping facial wounds and deep intra-oral wounds require an immediate referral to the local maxillofacial department. Extra-oral wounds should be secured with Steri-strips® prior to referral if possible.

### Intra-oral examination
- *Soft tissues*: To include thorough examination of all soft tissues including possible 'through and through' injuries, and injuries involving the floor of the mouth or tongue. Examine for swellings, lacerations, ecchymosis.
- *Bony hard tissues*: Check for steps/disruption on movements.
- *Dental hard tissues*:
  - *Chart teeth*: Account for all missing teeth/fragments.
  - *Chart*: Any fractures involving crown, crown-root or root.
  - *Note*: Mobility, displacement, reaction to percussion, occlusion, reaction to vitality tests.
- *Special tests*:
  - *Vitality*: Electric pulp test/ethyl chloride test.
  - *Radiographs*: At least two views to identify position/displacement and to diagnose injury (e.g. periapical and upper anterior occlusal or, two periapicals at different angles).
  - *Soft tissue radiographs*: If fragments are unaccounted for and there is related soft tissue injury.

**Table 7.1** Example of essential trauma chart.

| Tooth | 12 | 11 | 21 | 22 |
|---|---|---|---|---|
| EPT | Negative | Negative | 35 | 28 |
| Ethyl chloride | Negative | Negative | Positive | Positive |
| Mobility | Negative | Negative | Negative | Negative |
| TTP | Negative | Negative | Negative | Negative |
| Colour | Dark | Dark | Ok | Ok |
| Sinus | Negative | Negative | Negative | Negative |
| Radiograph | Apical root resorption | Apical radiolucency | Nil | Nil |

ETP, electric pulp test; TTP, tender to percussion.

## Management of traumatic dental injuries

### Management of soft tissue injuries

- Lavage (saline/chlorhexidine)
- Debridement of wound
- Arrest haemorrhage (direct pressure)
- Prescribe chlorhexidine mouthwash
- Where wound contamination or poor oral hygiene, antibiotics should be prescribed.

### Management of dental injuries

Management of injuries will be discussed as per diagnosis of injury to either the permanent or primary tooth and will be divided into immediate, intermediate and long-term follow-up. For all dental injuries, the patient should be advised to have a soft diet for a week, and to ensure the area is kept clean using 0.2% chlorhexidine mouthwash. This may help to prevent plaque accumulation and keep soft tissues healthy. In very young children, parents should be encouraged to keep the affected area clean using chlorhexidine mouthwash on gauze, if the child is unable to expectorate.

All dental/soft tissue injuries should be followed up and the essential trauma chart (Table 7.1) completed at each follow-up visit. This will ensure that any problems that may occur are identified early and can be dealt with in a timely manner.

## Injuries to the hard dental tissues and the pulp

### Enamel infraction

Enamel infraction relates to an incomplete fracture (crack) of the enamel without loss of tooth structure (see Figures 7.1 and 7.2).

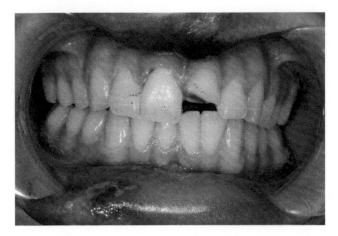

**Figure 7.1** Coronal fractures upper right lateral incisor (retained/fractured tooth fragment in place), upper right central incisor showing a star-shaped enamel infracture with embedded grit on the labial aspect and upper left central incisor showing a complicated crown fracture.

### Permanent dentition
#### *Immediate management*
- Result of investigations:
  - Visible fracture line
  - Not tender to percussion (TTP)
  - Normal mobility
  - Positive to vitality testing
  - No radiographic abnormalities (recommend periapical view)
- Treatment - no immediate treatment required

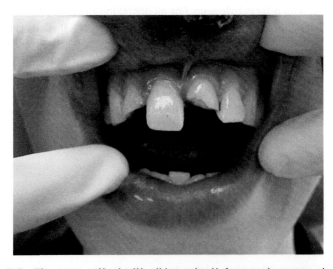

**Figure 7.2** The same patient with all loose tooth fragments removed. Complicated crown fractures confirmed on the upper right lateral incisor and upper left central incisor. Note the soft tissue injuries to the upper lip.

*Intermediate management*
Where marked infraction present, etch and seal with resin to prevent discolouration of the infraction lines.

*Follow-up*
No follow-up needed (unless associated with other dental injuries).

**Primary dentition**
As discussed in the preceding text for permanent dentition.

# Enamel fracture

A fracture confined to the enamel with loss of tooth structure.

## Permanent dentition
*Immediate management*
- Result of investigations:
  - Visible loss of enamel, no visible sign of exposed dentine
  - Not TTP
  - Normal mobility
  - Positive to vitality testing, if negative, monitor until definitive diagnosis
  - Radiographically, extent of tooth substance loss is visible
- Treatment (dependent on size of fracture):
  - If tooth fragment available, bond to tooth
  - Smooth sharp edges
  - Restore with composite resin

*Intermediate management*
- Investigations:
  - Radiograph at 6–8 weeks
- Treatment:
  - Not indicated

*Follow-up*
- Investigations:
  - Radiograph at 1 year

## Primary dentition
*Immediate management*
- Result of investigations:
  - Visible loss of enamel, no visible sign of exposed dentine
  - Not TTP
  - Normal mobility
  - Enamel loss visible radiographically
- Treatment:
  - Smooth sharp edges with Soflex® disc

### Intermediate management

- Investigations:
  - Review at 1 month, 3 months and 6 months
- Treatment:
  - No intermediate treatment indicated unless tooth become symptomatic

### Follow-up

- To review after every 4–6 months until exfoliation
- Radiograph if clinical signs are abnormal

## Enamel/dentine fracture

Enamel and dentine fractures with loss of tooth structure, but not involving the pulp.

### Permanent dentition
### Immediate management

- Result of investigations:
  - Visible loss of enamel and dentine, no visible sign of exposed pulp tissue
  - Not TTP
  - Normal mobility
  - Positive to vitality testing; if negative, monitor until definitive diagnosis
  - Radiographically, extent of tooth substance loss visible
  - Consider soft tissue radiograph if unable to locate lost tooth tissue
- Treatment:
  - Bond tooth fragment, if available.
  - If tooth fragment is not available, place a composite bandage (see below) or permanent composite restoration.
  - Composite bandage – cover exposed dentine with calcium hydroxide. Follow with etch, bond and placement of a light cured composite resin ensuring the whole fracture site is covered.

### Intermediate management

- Treatment:
  - Restoration with definitive composite material to restore function and aesthetics

### Follow-up

- Clinical and radiographic follow-up at 6–8 weeks and 1 year.

### Primary dentition
### Immediate management

- Result of investigations:
  - As discussed in the preceding text for permanent dentition, but no vitality testing

- Treatment:
  - Smooth sharp edges with a Soflex® disc
  - Restore subject to cooperation with composite material

### Follow-up
- Clinical and radiograph review at 6-8 weeks
- Radiograph if tooth becomes symptomatic, otherwise, monitor for asymptomatic exfoliation

## Enamel/dentine/pulp fracture

A fracture involving enamel and dentine with loss of tooth structure and exposure of the pulp.

### Permanent dentition
#### Immediate management
- Result of investigations:
  - Visible loss of enamel and dentine with exposed pulp tissue
  - Not usually tender to percussion
  - Normal mobility
  - Pulp usually sensitive to touch (If negative, has there been previous trauma?)
  - Radiographically, extent of tooth substance loss is visible
- Treatment:
  - In young patients with open apices (or even closed apices), attempt to preserve pulp vitality:
    - *Pulp capping*: Use in vital teeth with exposures less than 1 mm and less than 24 hours old:
      - With local anaesthetic and appropriate isolation, apply pulp-capping material (calcium hydroxide compound/ mineral trioxide aggregate (MTA)) to exposed pulp tissue. Ensure good seal over pulp cap with either re-bonding of tooth fragment or composite bandage.
    - *Partial pulpotomy*: Where exposure is minimal and less than 2 weeks old:
      - With local anaesthetic and under rubber dam, excise the coronal pulp tissue to a depth of 2 mm below the exposure site. Haemorrhage should be arrested with a clean cotton wool pledget and sterile water only. Apply non-setting calcium hydroxide, followed by setting calcium hydroxide calcium hydroxide over the healthy pulp tissue. Restore the tooth with composite. If haemorrhage continues after removal of the initial 2 mm of pulp tissue, this is indicative of necrotic tissue. A further 2 mm should be removed until healthy pulp tissue is reached. If this does not look achievable due to continuing haemorrhage, proceed to coronal pulpotomy.
    - *Coronal pulpotomy*: In vital teeth where exposure is large and greater than 2 weeks old:

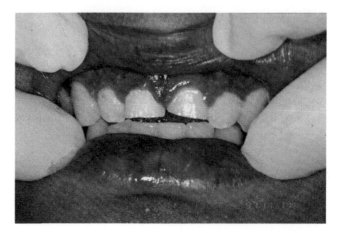

**Figure 7.3** Both upper central incisors with complicated crown fractures.

    ○ With local anaesthetic and under rubber dam, coronal pulp tissue should be excised to the level of the cervical constriction. Haemorrhage should be arrested with a clean cotton wool pledget and sterile water only. Apply 2–3 mm of non-setting calcium hydroxide, followed by setting calcium hydroxide. Restore tooth with composite restoration to ensure good seal (Figures 7.3 to 7.6).
    ○ In older patients with associated luxation injuries:
       ● Treatment of choice is extirpation and eventual root canal treatment.

### *Intermediate management*
● Treatment:
    ○ Ensure all definitive restorations have an excellent seal to avoid bacterial contamination of the pulp tissue.

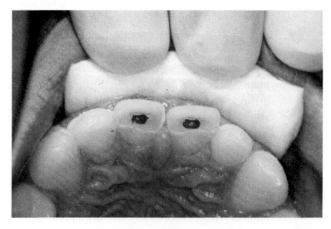

**Figure 7.4** Pulpotomies carried out on both upper permanent central incisor teeth.

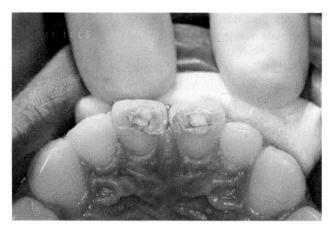

**Figure 7.5** Calcium hydroxide paste placed over healthy amputated pulp tissue.

### Follow-up

- Review appointments: At 1 month, 3 months, 6 months, 1 year, 18 months and 2 years.
  - If there are any signs of pathology, then the following should be done:
    - *Tooth with open apex*: Extirpation of necrotic pulp tissue and dress the root canal with non-setting calcium hydroxide. Achieve apexification with 3 monthly re-dresses using non-setting calcium hydroxide paste. Alternatively, place MTA at the open apex to achieve an artificial barrier. Eventually, definitive root filling once barrier achieved.
    - *Tooth with closed apex*: Extirpate necrotic pulp tissue and dress tooth with non-setting calcium hydroxide. On evidence of stabilisation of the pathology, a definitive root canal treatment can be placed.

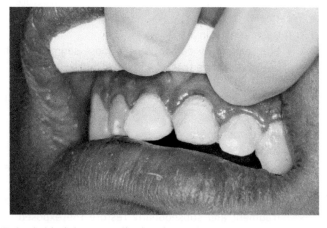

**Figure 7.6** Acid-etch composite 'bandage' placed to give hermetic seal.

### Primary dentition
#### Immediate management
- Result of investigations:
  - Visible loss of enamel and dentine with exposed pulp tissue
  - Not usually tender to percussion
  - Normal mobility
  - Radiographically, loss of tooth substance is visible
- Treatment:
  - Teeth with fractures into the pulp require extraction unless child can cooperate for pulp treatment.

#### Follow-up
- If pulp treatment performed, monitor at regular intervals to ensure asymptomatic and no signs of pathology.
- If extraction performed, monitor adjacent teeth for signs of pathology.

## Injuries to the hard dental tissues, the pulp and the alveolar process

### Crown-root fracture (uncomplicated)

A fracture involving enamel, dentine and cementum with loss of tooth structure, but not involving the pulp.

### Permanent dentition
#### Immediate management
- Result of investigations:
  - Visible crown fracture extending below the gingival margin
  - Tender to percussion
  - Coronal fragment appears mobile
  - Vitality testing usually positive for apical fragment
  - Radiographically, the apical extension of the fracture is hopefully visible
- Treatment:
  - If fragment still in place:
    - Stabilisation by cementing the loose segment to the adjacent teeth until a definitive treatment plan is made.
  - If fragment is lost:
    - Restore the exposed dentine above the gingival level with composite.

#### Intermediate management
- Treatment:
  - This depends on the clinical findings. These are several scenarios for restoring these teeth:
    - *Fragment removal only*: Remove the superficial coronal crown-root fragment and subsequently restore the exposed dentine above the gingival level with composite.

- *Fragment removal and post-crown placement*: The tooth will require root treatment. Fragment removal followed by obturation of the root canal. The tooth is then restored with a post and crown. In young children with complete apices, a fibre post and direct composite crown build up can be placed using a crown-forma.
- *Orthodontic extrusion of apical fragment*: Once root canal treatment has been completed, perform orthodontic extrusion of the remaining root to a sufficient length to enable restoration to be completed with a post-crown.
- *Surgical extrusion*: Remove the fractured tooth fragment and subsequent surgical repositioning of the root into a more coronal position. Splint flexibly for 6–8 weeks. Once periodontal healing ensues, complete definitive restoration with a crown build up.
- *Decoronation*: This is where future treatment plan involves implant placement. The root is left in situ to maintain bone levels and avoid alveolar bone resorption. This leaves a more optimum site for later implant placement. Interim treatment would involve construction of a partial denture to act as a space maintainer and maintain aesthetics.
- *Extraction*: This is inevitable with very deep crown-root fractures or vertical fractures where a definitive restoration is impossible.

### Follow-up
- All the treatment modalities have their advantages and disadvantages. Some treatment options may be better referred for treatment to be completed in a specialist centre. Prognosis of traumatised teeth will not be influenced by a delay of treatment within a time frame of 1–2 weeks.
- Teeth should be monitored at intervals of 1, 3, 6, 12, 18 months to 2 years.
- Radiographs should be taken at the time of trauma, 6 and 18 months post-operatively (and at relevant stages of root canal treatment).

## Primary dentition
### Immediate management
- Result of investigations:
  - As discussed in the preceding text for permanent dentition but omitting the vitality testing. Crown-root fractures are unusual in primary teeth.
- Treatment:
  - Treatment of choice for primary teeth is extraction.
  - Warn patient/parent of potential damage to permanent successor teeth.

### Follow-up
- Monitor adjacent teeth for signs of pathology.
- Monitor for asymptomatic eruption of secondary dentition.

## Crown-root fracture (complicated)

A fracture involving the enamel, dentine and cementum with loss of tooth structure and involving the pulp.

### Permanent dentition
#### *Immediate management*
- Result of investigations:
  - Visible crown fracture extending below the gingival margin (crown fragment may be lost)
  - Tender to percussion
  - Coronal fragment mobile
  - Apical fragment usually tests positive to vitality testing
  - Radiographically, apical extension of fracture usually not visible on standard periapical view (suggest periapical and occlusal radiographs)
- Treatment:
  - *If fragment in place*: Temporary stabilisation of loose segments to adjacent teeth until definitive diagnosis can be made.
  - *If fragment lost*: Extirpate pulp, dress with non-setting calcium hydroxide and place temporary restoration.
  - *Young patients*: Optimum is to maintain pulp vitality in teeth with open apices by completing a partial pulpotomy. This is also the choice for young children with complete apices. Suitable materials include MTA or calcium hydroxide compounds.
  - *In older patients*: Root canal treatment is the treatment of choice.

#### *Intermediate management*
- Determine definitive treatment depending on clinical findings.
- Many of these options can be deferred for later treatment and are best referred for treatment in specialist settings.
- Treatment options:
  - *Fragment removal and gingivectomy*: Removal of loose fragment, subsequent endodontic treatment and restoration with a post-retained crown. A gingivectomy may need to be performed prior to placement of a definitive restoration.
  - *Orthodontic extrusion of apical fragment*: Removal of the loose fragment, subsequent endodontic treatment and orthodontic extrusion of the remaining root with sufficient length after extrusion to support a post-retained crown.
  - *Surgical extrusion*: Removal of the fractured fragment with repositioning of the root in a more coronal position. Splint tooth in new position.
  - *Decoronation*: If an implant solution is planned, the root fragment may be left in situ after total crown removal in order to avoid alveolar resorption and therefore maintaining the volume of the alveolar process for later optimal implant placement.

○ *Extraction*: Inevitably the choice for very deep crown-root fractures, the extreme being a vertical fracture.

### Follow-up
- Clinical and radiographic reviews at regular intervals dependent on treatment completed.
- Monitor for signs of pathology, including resorption.

## Primary dentition
### Immediate management
- Result of investigations:
  ○ As discussed in the preceding text for permanent dentition, but no vitality testing
- Treatment:
  ○ Extraction

### Intermediate/Follow-up
- Monitor adjacent teeth for signs of pathology.
- Monitor for asymptomatic eruption of secondary dentition.

# Root fracture

A fracture involving cementum, dentine and the pulp. Can be classified by whether the coronal fragment is displaced or not.

## Permanent dentition
### Immediate management
- Result of investigations:
  ○ Visually, the coronal segment may be mobile, and in some cases, displaced.
  ○ Tooth may be tender.
  ○ Vitality testing may initially give negative results, monitor until definitive diagnosis made.
  ○ Radiographically, root fracture line usually visible. This may appear in a horizontal or diagonal plane (ideal radiographic view would be an upper anterior occlusal).
- Treatment:
  ○ Under local anaesthetic, reposition the coronal fragment using digital manipulation.
  ○ A splint (e.g. composite and orthodontic wire) should be used to stabilise the loose fragment for 4 weeks.
  ○ The splint should be placed to involve at least one tooth on either side of the traumatised tooth.
  ○ Teeth with cervical fractures require a longer healing time, and it is indicated to leave the splint on for a period of up to 4 months.

### Intermediate management
- Treatment:
  - o For apical/mid-third root fractures – after 4 weeks, remove the splint and assess the tooth.
  - o For cervical third root fractures – after a period of up to 4 months, remove the splint and assess the tooth. If still mobile, re-splint for a further 2 weeks.
  - o Root canal treatment may be commenced at any stage during the monitoring process where there are symptoms of pulpal necrosis – negative response to vitality testing (electrical/thermal), discolouration and evidence of a *radiolucency adjacent to the fracture line*.
  - o Root canal treatment should be completed by dressing the tooth with non-setting calcium hydroxide *to the level of the fracture line*. The purpose is to attain a calcific barrier at this level and leave the untreated apical root fragment in situ, without intervention. Where the apical fragment requires removal, this may be completed by apicectomy.

### Follow-up
- Healing should be monitored for up to 1 year post-trauma.
- Clinical and radiographic assessment at 6–8 weeks, 4 months post-trauma (Note that for cervical third fractures, the splint may be removed at this time).
- Further reviews should take place at 6 months, 1 year and yearly for 5 years.

## Primary dentition
### Immediate management
- Result of investigations – as discussed in the preceding text for permanent dentition, but without the vitality testing.
- Treatment:
  - o Extract the loose coronal fragment carefully. The apical fragments may be left in situ to resorb, rather than attempting removal with elevators and causing potential damage to the permanent successor.

### Follow-up
- Warn patient/parents of potential damage to the underlying permanent successor.

# Injuries to the periodontal tissues

## Concussion/subluxation

An injury to the tooth supporting structures resulting in increased mobility but without displacement of the tooth. With subluxation injuries, bleeding from the gingival crevice is evident.

### Permanent dentition
*Immediate management*
- Result of investigations:
  - Visually, no displacement.
  - Tooth is tender to percussion.
  - No increased mobility of tooth.
  - Usually, a positive vitality test. If negative vitality test, monitor until definitive diagnosis.
  - Radiographically, no abnormalities noted (tooth in situ in the socket).
- Treatment:
  - No immediate treatment required.
  - With subluxation injuries: Splint for up to 2 weeks for patient comfort.

*Intermediate management*
- Treatment:
  - Monitor pulpal condition for 1 year post-trauma.
  - If signs of pulpal necrosis (unlikely), carry out root canal treatment.

*Follow-up*
- Clinical and radiographic assessment at 4, 6–8 weeks and 1 year post-trauma.

### Primary dentition
*Immediate management*
- Result of investigations:
  - As discussed in the preceding text for permanent dentition, but no vitality testing advised.
- Treatment:
  - No immediate treatment required.

*Follow-up*
- Monitor as discussed previously (no further radiographs unless symptomatic).

## Extrusion

A partial displacement of the tooth out of its socket, leaving the alveolar bone intact. This results in partial or total separation of the periodontal ligament resulting in loosening and displacement of the tooth.

### Permanent dentition
*Immediate management*
- Result of investigations:
  - Visually, the tooth appears elongated
  - Tender to percussion

- o Excessively mobile
- o Vitality testing may be inconclusive
- Treatment:
  - o Clean the exposed root surface with saline prior to repositioning.
  - o Reposition the tooth by gently pushing it back into the tooth socket with axial digital pressure (with or without local anaesthetic).
  - o Place a splint for 2 weeks.

### Intermediate management

- Treatment:
  - o Monitor the pulpal condition in order to diagnose associated root resorption:
    - *Open apex*: The aim is to monitor for revascularisation by looking for signs of continued root formation, pulpal canal obliteration and positive vitality testing. Monitor for signs of pulpal necrosis.
    - *Closed apex*: A continued lack of pulp response to vitality testing indicated pulpal necrosis, together with periapical pathology radiographically and crown discolouration.
  - o Where signs of pulpal necrosis, begin pulp extirpation and root canal treatment. In teeth with open apices, apexification will be necessary prior to definitive obturation.

### Follow-up

- Clinical and radiographical assessment and splint removal after 2 weeks. Assess for pulpal vitality/continued dental development at 4 weeks, 6-8 weeks, 6 months and 1 year.

### Primary dentition
### Immediate management

- Result of investigations:
  - o As discussed in the preceding text for permanent dentition, but without vitality testing.
- Treatment:
  - o Dependent on extent of extrusion:
    - If loose (danger of inhaling) or patient cannot close mouth or eat – extraction.
    - If minimal to monitor

## Lateral luxation

Displacement of the tooth other than axially. Displacement is accompanied by comminution or fracture of either the labial or the palatal/lingual alveolar bone. Often, the tooth has been forced into the bone by displacement and the tooth frequently appears firm.

## Permanent dentition
### *Immediate management*
- Result of investigations:
  - Tooth visibly appears displaced, usually in a palatal/lingual or labial direction.
  - On percussion, tooth gives a high metallic (ankylotic) sound.
  - Usually locked solid in the bone.
  - Except in cases where there are minor displacements, tooth will give a negative response to vitality testing.
  - Radiographically, there appears to be a widened periodontal ligament space. Best radiographic view would be an occlusal view.
- Treatment:
  - Give local anaesthesia.
  - Reposition the tooth with forceps or with digital pressure to ensure it is disengaged from its bony lock. Gently reposition the tooth into its original location.
  - Stabilise the tooth with a splint for 4 weeks.
  - Where evidence of an open wound/laceration, chlorhexidine mouthwash and antibiotics should be prescribed.

### *Intermediate management*
- Treatment:
  - As discussed in Section 'Extrusion'.

### *Follow-up*
- As discussed in Section 'Extrusion'.

## Primary dentition-
### *Immediate management*
- Result of investigations:
  - As discussed in the preceding text for permanent dentition, but without the vitality testing.
- Treatment:
  - Depends on the direction of the luxation:
    - *Palatal crown luxations*: Where the apex has been displaced labially, away from the developing tooth germ, no treatment required (as long as the crown is not in traumatic occlusion). Over the next 1–2 months the tongue will often reposition the affected tooth.
    - *Buccal crown displacement*: It is rare. The apex of the primary tooth is displaced towards the developing tooth germ and treatment of choice is extraction.

### *Intermediate management*
- Treatment:
  - If the tooth has been left in situ, monitor for spontaneous repositioning.

    o If any signs of pulpal necrosis during the review period, treatment of choice is extraction.

### Follow-up
- Advise the parents to look for signs of infection when brushing the child's teeth.
- To look for signs of colour change, tenderness while eating, swelling above the affected tooth.
- Review tooth at 1 week, 1, 3, 6 months and then every 4-6 months at check-up appointments. Radiographs should be taken at the time of trauma, 3 months later and at any sign of pathology appearing.

## Intrusion- open apex/closed apex

Displacement of the tooth into the alveolar bone. This injury is accompanied by fracture of the alveolar socket.

### Permanent dentition
#### Immediate management
- Result of investigations:
  - o The tooth is visibly displaced axially in to the alveolar bone.
  - o On percussion, a high 'metallic' (ankylotic) sound is noted.
  - o No mobility.
  - o Negative to vitality testing (unless minor displacement).
  - o Radiographically, periodontal ligament space may be absent from all or part of the root.
- Treatment:
  - o This depends on the severity of the intrusion and the maturity of the tooth as follows:
    - Open apex (6-11 yr) and intrusion up to 7 mm:
      - o Allow for spontaneous eruption. This injury has excellent eruptive potential.
    - Intrusion more than 7 mm:
      - o As discussed in the preceding text for intrusion up to 7 mm.
    - Closed apex (12-17 yr) and intrusion up to 7 mm:
      - o As given in the preceding text for intrusion up to 7 mm.
    - Intrusion more than 7 mm (12-17 yr) and intrusion up to and more than 7 mm (>17 yr):
      - o *Orthodontic repositioning*: Clean the area. Adapt steel arch wire to anterior region. Apply orthodontic brackets to anterior region with elastic traction. Monitor for 10 days to assess orthodontic extrusion of tooth (if no progress, move to surgical repositioning).
      - o *Surgical repositioning*: Indicated when major dislocation of tooth (approximately more than half crown length). Under local anaesthesia, reposition with forceps. Clean the area. Suture laceration if present

and apply a splint for 4 weeks. Splint removal and radiographs 4 weeks post-trauma.
  - o *Patient instructions*: Soft diet for 1 week and to keep good oral hygiene.

### Intermediate management
- Treatment:
  - o Severe intrusion injuries can often result in root resorption.
  - o The risk of resorption can be minimised by initiating root canal treatment in all cases with completed root formation, and where chances of pulp revascularisation is unlikely.
  - o Root canal treatment should start 3–4 weeks post-trauma.
  - o The canal should be dressed with non-setting calcium hydroxide paste and changed every 3 months until there is evidence that no root resorption is taking place.

### Follow-up
- Clinical and radiographic assessment at 6–8 weeks, 6 months, 1 year and yearly for 5 years.

## Primary dentition
### Immediate management
- Result of investigations:
  - o Assess the displacement of the traumatised tooth root to see where the root lies in relation to the permanent successor. If the root lies buccally, this should ensure the underlying tooth remains unharmed.
  - o Radiographically, an upper anterior occlusal radiograph is ideal.
- Treatment:
  - o No treatment necessary, to monitor for spontaneous re-eruption.

### Intermediate management
- Investigations:
  - o Monitor for visible signs of non-vitality, to include colour change, swelling above the affected tooth and/or tenderness when eating.
- Treatment:
  - o If any signs of infection – extract.

### Follow-up
- *Partial intrusion*: If no re-eruption at 4 months, leave in situ and monitor closely for normal resorption and exfoliation (given no signs of infection).
- *Complete intrusion*: If no significant re-eruption after 4–6 months (no signs of movement), then consider surgical removal dependent on age of patient and possibility of intruded tooth causing delayed eruption of permanent successor.

- *Where tooth is being monitored and extraction not planned*:
  - ○ Clinical assessment at 1 week, then monthly until 6 months post-trauma. Thereafter, monitor at every 6 monthly assessment.
  - ○ Radiograph 3 months post-trauma and at any other time there are clinical signs of non-vitality.

## Avulsion

The tooth is completely displaced out of its socket.

### Permanent dentition

Ensure the tooth is permanent. Do not replant primary teeth. Immediate advice if required over the phone:

- Find the tooth and pick it up by the crown ('the white part'). Avoid touching the root.
- If the tooth is dirty, wash it briefly under cold running water.
- Replant tooth in socket and try to get the patient to bite on a handkerchief to hold it in position.
- If the patient is unable to have the tooth replanted, place it in a glass of milk.
- Seek emergency dental treatment immediately.

### *Immediate management*

- Result of investigations:
  - ○ The tooth is absent from its socket. There may be evidence of coagulum in the socket.
  - ○ No further tests required, except radiographs where suspicion of intrusion, root fracture, alveolar fracture or jaw fracture.
  - ○ Upper anterior occlusal radiograph is ideal.
- Check:
  - ○ The time the tooth is out of the mouth, extra-alveolar time (EAT) and extra-alveolar dry time (EADT).
  - ○ The method of storage (wet or dry).
  - ○ Any contamination.
  - ○ Was the tooth rinsed, and if so, with what?
  - ○ Any relevant medical history (including tetanus status).
- Treatment:
  - ○ This is dependent on the maturity of the tooth (open or closed apex Figures 7.7, 7.8 and 7.9), how the tooth is stored prior to arrival at the dental clinic and patient cooperation.
  - ○ Delayed replantation has a poor long-term prognosis. The periodontal ligament will be necrotic and cannot be expected to heal. The goal in doing delayed replantation is to preserve alveolar bone. The expected eventual outcome is ankylosis and resorption of the root.
  - ○ In patients where growth is not complete, when ankylosis occurs, infraposition of the tooth may also occur. When the infraposition of the tooth crown is more than 1 mm, it is recommended to perform decoronation to preserve the contour of the alveolar ridge.

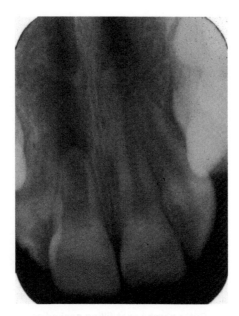

**Figure 7.7** Upper right permanent central incisor showing a non-vital tooth with arrested root development and an immature, open apex.

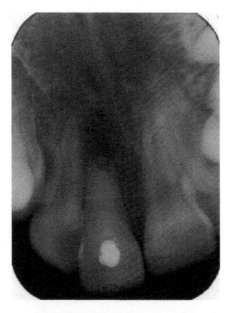

**Figure 7.8** Intra-canal dressing with radiopaque calcium hydroxide paste, which completely fills the root canal. At 2 months.

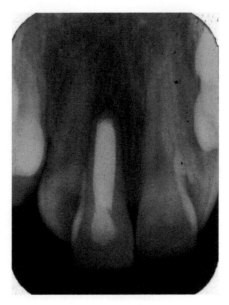

**Figure 7.9**  Gutta percha root filling packed against an apical barrier. At 10 months.

Management of avulsed teeth in specific scenarios is summarised in Table 7.2.

### Primary dentition
#### *Immediate management*
- Result of investigations:
  - No further tests required, except radiographs where suspicion of intrusion, root fracture, alveolar fracture, or jaw fracture.
- Treatment:
  - No further treatment necessary. Do not replant primary teeth.

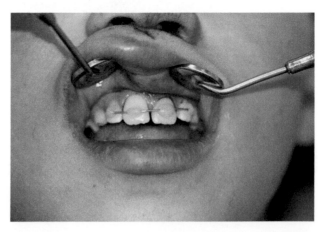

**Figure 7.10**  Upper left central incisor avulsed, replanted and splinted with a simple composite/wire splint.

**Table 7.2** Management regimens for avulsed teeth.

| Status of tooth | Treatment | Follow-up |
|---|---|---|
| Closed apex: Tooth replanted prior to patients arrival at dental surgery | Leave tooth in situ<br>Clean the area<br>Check replanted tooth in correct position clinically and radiographically<br>Splint flexibly for 1–2 wk (Figure 7.10)<br>Prescribe antibiotics<br>Check tetanus status | Clinical assessment weekly for the first month<br>Root canal treatment 7–10 d post-trauma<br>Place calcium hydroxide paste for 1 mo and check for pathology prior to final obturation<br>Remove splint and assess (clinical and radiographic control at 4 wk, 3 mo, 6 mo, 1 yr and yearly thereafter) |
| Closed apex: EADT<60 min tooth stored in appropriate storage medium | Clean tooth with sterile water<br>Irrigate socket with sterile water<br>Replant tooth with gentle pressure<br>Check replanted tooth in correct position clinically and radiographically<br>Splint flexibly for 1–2 wk<br>Prescribe antibiotics<br>Check tetanus status | Clinical assessment weekly for the first month<br>Root canal treatment 7–10 d post-replantation<br>Place calcium hydroxide paste for 1 mo and check for pathology prior to final obturation<br>Remove splint and assess (clinical and radiographic) after 1–2 wk<br>Clinical and radiograph control at 4 wk, 3 mo, 6 mo, 1 yr and yearly thereafter |
| Closed apex: EADT >60 min or longer storage in non-physiological media | Poor long-term prognosis<br>Remove attached soft tissue with gauze<br>Irrigate with saline<br>Replant tooth with gentle pressure<br>Check replanted tooth in correct position clinically and radiographically<br>Splint flexibly for 4 wk to achieve ankylosis<br>Prescribe antibiotics<br>Check tetanus status | Clinical assessment weekly for the first month<br>Root canal treatment 7–10 d post-trauma<br>Remove splint and assess (clinical and radiographic) after 4 wk<br>Clinical and radiograph control at 4 wk, 3 mo, 6 mo, 1 yr and yearly thereafter |

*(continued)*

**Table 7.2** Management regimens for avulsed teeth (*continued*).

| Status of tooth | Treatment | Follow-up |
|---|---|---|
| Open apex:<br>Tooth replanted prior to the patients arrival at the dental surgery | Leave the tooth in situ<br>Clean the area<br>Check replanted tooth in correct position clinically and radiographically<br>Splint flexibly for 1–2 wk<br>Prescribe antibiotics<br>Check tetanus status | Clinical assessment weekly for the first month<br>Remove splint and assess (clinical and radiographic) after 2 wk<br>Root canal treatment should be avoided unless there is clinical and/or radiographic evidence of pulp necrosis<br>Clinical and radiograph control at 4 wk, 3 mo, 6 mo, 1 yr and yearly thereafter |
| Open apex:<br>EADT < 60 min tooth stored in appropriate storage medium | Irrigate socket with saline<br>Replant tooth with gentle pressure<br>Check replanted tooth in correct position clinically and radiographically<br>Splint flexibly for up to 2 wk<br>Prescribe antibiotics<br>Check tetanus status | Clinical assessment weekly for the first month<br>Remove splint and assess (clinical and radiographic) after 2 wk<br>Root canal treatment should be avoided unless there is clinical and/or radiographic evidence of pulp necrosis<br>Clinical and radiograph control at 4 wk, 3 mo, 6 mo, 1 yr and yearly thereafter |
| Open apex:<br>EADT>60 min or longer storage in non-physiological media | Poor long-term prognosis<br>Immerse the tooth in a 2% sodium fluoride solution for 20 min<br>Irrigate with saline<br>Replant tooth with gentle pressure<br>Check replanted tooth in correct position clinically and radiographically<br>Splint flexibly for 1 wk only to try to avoid ankylosis<br>Prescribe antibiotics<br>Check tetanus status | Root canal treatment 7–10 d post-trauma with splint in place<br>Remove splint<br>Assess (clinical and radiographic) after 4 wk<br>Clinical and radiograph control at 3 mo, 6 mo, 1 yr and yearly thereafter |

EADT, extra-alveolar dry time.

## Dento-alveolar fractures

Dento-alveolar fractures are said to have occurred when the tooth-bearing part of the mandible or maxilla is involved in the injury. If there is minimal mobility and displacement of the fracture these injuries are often managed conservatively, particularly when the dental occlusion is normal. It is often useful to prescribe a short course of antibiotics if the mucosal integrity is breached.

Cases of non-surgical management include the following:

- Minimal or no displacement of the fracture
- Normal occlusion
- Minimal or no soft or hard tissue loss
- No bleeding or likelihood of infection if untreated
- A cooperative patient

Conservative management involves advice about a soft diet and oral hygiene. Regular follow-up of such patients is required. It is important that if the situation changes, for example evidence of infection developing, that this is treated effectively.

### Surgical management of dento-alveolar fractures

The principles of open reduction and internal fixation using plates can often be applied in these situations but much depends on the size of the bone fragments and an inventive approach often needs to be taken. Sometimes, splinting the teeth using orthodontic brackets as aforementioned will be sufficient to stabilise the dento-alveolar segment. When operating on dento-alveolar fractures, the possibility of compromising the blood supply to the area should be minimised.

If the bony segment is badly comminuted or there is significant soft tissue loss leading to poor supply to the fragment, on occasion judicious removal of bone fragments may be required, but great care must be exercised in such situations.

Treatment of fractured teeth attached to the dento-alveolar fragment may be carried out at the same time but removal of teeth is sometimes carried out as a secondary procedure to maximise the stability of the segment, particularly with regard to its blood supply.

## Conclusions

The clinician working in a dental emergency clinic will encounter patients with traumatised teeth and supporting structures. Specific situations require different treatment regimens. It is important in all cases not to lose sight of the fact that the patient should be seen as a whole, both from the point of view of possible concomitant head injury or injuries to other parts of the body.

## Further reading

Andreasen JO, Andreasen FM, Andersson L (eds) (2007) *Textbook and Color Atlas of Traumatic Injuries to the Teeth*, 4th edn. Wiley-Blackwell, Oxford.

# Chapter 8
# Pain Relief in the Dental Emergency Clinic

## U.J. Moore

This chapter discusses the following:

- The mechanism of pain
- Dental causes of pain
- Management of pain symptoms
- Analgesic preparations

## Introduction

In a dental emergency clinic, pain is one of the most common causes for patient attendance. Practitioners should understand how pain is generated and how best to control it.

As a general principle, it must be remembered that the best form of analgesia is to remove the underlying cause that is leading to pain. Some hints on the drugs to prescribe and the choices available are given later in this chapter.

## General mechanism of pain

Pain is a powerful motivating force for all sensate beings. It is described as 'an unpleasant sensory and emotional experience associated with actual or potential tissue damage'. The sensory nervous system alerts an organism to any noxious stimuli that it might be in contact with and often sets off a reflex withdrawal from the source of pain. Awareness of sensation is vital to survival and pain is the most emotionally charged of all sensations. Thus, there is also a strong psychological and therefore subjective element to an individual's response to any painful situation.

*Dental Emergencies*, First Edition. Edited by Mark Greenwood and Ian Corbett.
© 2012 Blackwell Publishing Ltd. Published 2012 by Blackwell Publishing Ltd.

**Table 8.1** Speed of conduction and activity of nerve fibres.

| Nerve fibres | Speed of conduction | Activity |
|---|---|---|
| Aβ – myelinated | 35–120 m/s | Touch, proprioception |
| Aδ – myelinated | 5–30 m/s | Pain |
| C – unmyelinated | 0.4–1 m/s | Pain |

Nerve fibres subserving pain, touch and proprioception are shown in Table 8.1. They react to a large number of mediators, most of which are involved in the inflammatory response. These mediators, when released during tissue damage from whatever cause, stimulate the pain fibres that conduct stimuli centrally. Repetitive stimulation can cause a state of central sensitisation, which makes further stimulation give rise to more prolonged pain perception.

The initial stimulus may not be perceived as pain as there is thought to be a gate control mechanism, first described by Wall and Melzack. This 'gate' is a synaptic link between the initial impulse and the central connections leading to the perception of pain (Figure 8.1). A single pain impulse may not pass through this gate, but if the stimuli are sufficient, pain will be perceived. Other sensory fibres (Aβ) transmit stimuli more rapidly than pain fibres and impulses also pass into and through this gate mechanism. These other impulses are thought to modulate the opening and closing of the gate against pain stimuli and this results in the possibility of blocking pain by closing the gate due to overload from other sensory stimuli, such as pressure. This phenomenon is described as afferent inhibition.

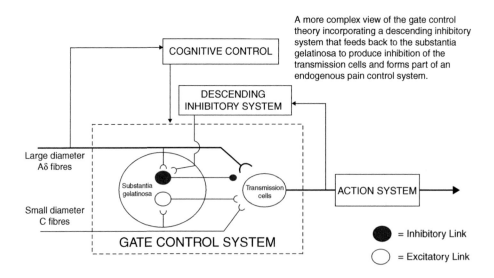

**Figure 8.1** Modified gate control mechanism (Melzack and Wall, 1982).

## Pain types

Three main types of pain are described as follows:

(1) *Nociception*: It arises as a result of the inflammatory response in tissue injury.
(2) *Neuropathic pain*: It is due to an altered neural response, often as a result of damage, such as post-herpetic neuralgia but may arise spontaneously, as in trigeminal neuralgia.
(3) *Psychogenic pain*: The category in which atypical facial pain falls. Such pain often causes chronic symptoms requiring very careful management.

## Pain/inflammatory mediators

There are a large number of pain mediators. Such mediators can act singly or together to intensify the perception of pain. Many of the mediators are involved in other aspects of the inflammatory response, such as increasing vascular permeability. With an increase in the inflammatory response, the site of damage can become either hyperalgesic, when any stimulus is perceived as pain, or there may be peripheral sensitisation in which pain thresholds are lowered, giving rise to more afferent nociceptive activity. Some of the more important mediators are outlined in Sections 'Peripheral mediators and Central mediators'. A more comprehensive list is included in Tables 8.2 and 8.3.

### Peripheral mediators

- *Prostaglandins*: These are a family of phospholipids generated from arachidonic acid, derived from cell walls, by the action of cyclooxygenase. These are powerful mediators of pain and it is principally the action of non-steroidal analgesics on prostaglandin synthesis by inhibition of cyclooxygenase that gives rise to their analgesic effects (Figures 8.2 and 8.3).
- *Bradykinins*: These are linked to plasma kininogen.
- *Serotonin*: It is derived from platelets.
- *Histamine*: It is released from mast cells that are ruptured during tissue damage.
- *Leukotrienes*: These are derived from arachidonic acid by the action of lipoxygenase and are linked to histamine production.

The inhibition of these mediators is the principal action of most peripherally acting analgesics.

### Central mediators

An even larger number of central nervous system transmitters involved in the perception of pain have been isolated. However, *substance P* has been shown to be involved in the mechanism of pain both centrally and peripherally. Opioid action through the *endorphin system* may, in part, be due to its activity against

**Table 8.2** Peripheral inflammatory mediators. The main peripheral mediators involved in the inflammatory response that seem to generate pain stimuli. Non-steroidal anti-inflammatory drugs only seem to influence prostaglandin synthesis.

| Mediator | Chemistry | Distribution | Actions |
|---|---|---|---|
| Prostaglandins $PGE_2$ $PGI_2$ $TA_2$ | Derived from arachidonic acid by cyclooxygenase | $PGE_2$, $PGI_2$ cell membrane Found in inflamed tissue $TA_2$ from platelets | Vasodilatation, hyperalgesia Sensitise nerve ending to other mediators $TA_2$ cause platelet aggregation |
| Leukotrienes LTB4 LTD4 | Derived from arachidonic acid by lipoxygenase | Cell membrane phospholipid Found in inflamed tissue | Hyperalgesia Synthesis of prostaglandins and substance P |
| Platelet activating factor (PAF) | Phospholipid | Released from leucocytes and platelets | Causes platelet aggregation, release of $TA_2$ vasodilatation, chemotactic, hyperalgesia |
| Kinins Bradykinin | Peptides Nonapeptide | Blood and tissue fluids, increased in inflammation | Potent pain producer Activates other mediators |
| 5-Hydroxy-tryptamine Serotonin | Amino acid | Platelets in man | Vasodilatation through $PGE_2$ Pain when applied to blister base |
| Histamine | Amino acid | Mast cells due to tissue injury, action of bradykinin and substance P | Vasodilatation co-mediator |
| Substance P | Peptide | Released from nerve endings | Peripheral nerve transmission Vasodilatation, strong flare and itch reaction |

substance P, but a larger part might be the modulation of the effects of pain rather than modifying the stimulus itself. Endogenous opioid receptors can change the way in which pain is perceived. Table 8.3 contains a summary of central transmitters.

In summary, peripherally acting analgesics seem to have efficacy by reducing stimulation of pain fibres by suppressing the release or synthesis of

**Table 8.3** Central transmitters. Some commonly used peripherally acting analgesics. For more information about dosages, always consult the British National Formulary.

| Transmitter | Chemistry | Distribution | Actions |
|---|---|---|---|
| Endorphins<br>Enkephalins<br>Dynorphins | Peptides<br>Peptides<br>Peptides | Arcuate nuclei<br>Thalamus,<br>brainstem<br>Throughout CNS<br>Hypothalamus<br>Limbic system,<br>brainstem | Post-synaptic<br>inhibition<br>of neurones or<br>presynaptic<br>inhibition of<br>transmitter<br>release |
| Substance P | Polypeptide<br>(Undecapep-<br>tide) | Central terminal of<br>dorsal root | Enhances C-fibre<br>activity.<br>Interaction between<br>substance P and<br>enkephalins |
| 5-HT<br>(5-hydroxy-<br>tryptamine<br>serotonin) | Amine | Platelets<br>Superficial layers of<br>dorsal horn | Inhibition and<br>excitation.<br>Influence on opioid<br>analgesia |
| ATP (adenosine<br>triphosphate) | Purines | Spinal cord primary<br>afferents | Contribution to<br>spinal action of<br>opioid suppression<br>of transmission of<br>sensory information |
| VIP (vasoactive<br>intestinal<br>peptide) | Amino acid | Afferent pathways<br>of spinal cord | Suggested<br>involvement in pain<br>transmission |
| Cholecystokinin | Peptide | Brain and spinal<br>cord | Unclear |
| Amino acids<br>GABA<br>(inhibitory)<br>Glutamate<br>(excitatory) | Amino acid<br>Amino acid | Periaqueductal grey<br>Nucleus raphe<br>magnus<br>Nucleus<br>gigantocellularis<br>Universal | Analgesia in man<br>Excitation of dorsal<br>horn cells |
| Catecholamines<br>Dopamine<br>Adrenaline<br>Noradrenaline | Derived from<br>phenylalanine<br>and tyrosine | Basal ganglia<br>Hypothalamus<br>Amygdala,<br>Hippocampus<br>Medullary reticular<br>formation | Probably inhibitory<br>Suppression of<br>afferent evoked<br>activity in dorsal<br>horn<br>Not clear |

CNS, central nervous system; tds, three times daily; qds, four times daily, GABA, gamma-aminobutyric acid.

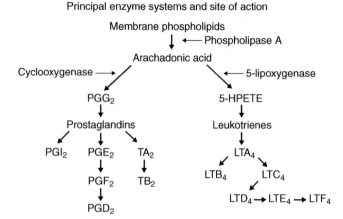

**Figure 8.2** Synthesis of arachidonic acid derivatives.

mediators at the site of the noxious stimulus. Centrally acting analgesics may alter the response of these stimuli as they arrive centrally, by blockade of conduction or alteration of perception of the stimulus as pain.

## Distribution of pain fibres in the mouth and jaws

The sensory nerve supply to the mouth, teeth and jaws is entirely from the maxillary and mandibular divisions of the trigeminal nerve. Some areas encountered far back in the mouth and tongue are supplied by the glossopharyngeal nerve, but this is rarely of significance in the management of dental pain.

The teeth have a very rich supply of sensation, with the pulp only having pain fibres within it. This means that all sensation in the pulp is perceived as painful,

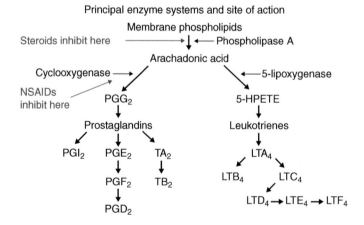

**Figure 8.3** Sites of inhibition of prostaglandin synthesis.

either from noxious products of inflammation, or increased pressure within the closed pulp chamber. This may help to explain the intransigent and constant nature of pulpal pain as the gate control mechanism only receives pain stimuli and thus will only act as an open gate in this situation. It may also explain why pulpal pain is so difficult to control with peripherally acting analgesics alone. Once damage to pulp causes irreversible pulpitis, the circulation to the pulp is compromised and thus pain fibres have no chance of relief until pulpal necrosis takes place with consequent death of pulp and associated pain fibres. All other areas of the body have other sensory supplies such as pressure and proprioception that can influence the gate control mechanism. All these elements in the jaws are found in the periodontal ligament rather than within the teeth.

## Sources of pain in the mouth and jaws

### Organic causes of pain

- *Inflammation*: Pulpitis.
- *Trauma (physical, chemical)*: Many situations can contribute to the traumatic aspect of pain, apart from obvious direct blows, such as clenching, grinding, sudden excessive biting forces as when biting an unexpected hard object, habitual nail-biting, cheek-biting, and so forth. Chemical insults may include direct application of acidic or caustic compounds to the oral tissues.
- *Infection*: This is by the far the commonest cause of pain in the mouth and is usually of dental origin. Infections in other sites, such as salivary glands, occur but much less frequently. Most types of micro-organism can be implicated in oral infection with bacteria, fungae and viruses being commonly represented.
- *Foreign body*: This is relatively unusual but foreign bodies may be introduced under ill-fitting dentures or by deliberate implantation of 'foreign' material such as dressings to sockets.
- *Autoimmune*: Autoimmune disease can affect the oral tissues, most commonly to cause painful ulceration.
- *Neuropathic*: Neuralgic pain can affect the mouth. Most commonly, this is in the form of trigeminal neuralgia that arises as a result of trauma, viral infection or intra-cranial nerve compression. The pain is described as a sudden, usually unilateral, severe, brief, stabbing, recurrent pain in the distribution of one or more branches of the fifth cranial nerve (see Chapter 6). Post-herpetic neuralgia is also encountered as a separate disease process.
- *Unknown*: Some disease processes, such as lichen planus, have no clearly identifiable cause, and controlling symptoms is the main aim of treatment.
- *Neoplasia*: Pain is not necessarily an early manifestation of neoplasia in the mouth but can certainly affect later stages of the disease process.

### Psychogenic – non-organic causes of pain

See Section 'Psychogenic – non-organic causes of pain'.

## Control of pain

Simply stated, the choices for the clinician revolve around:

- controlling local tissue damage and release of inflammatory mediators;
- blockade of nociceptive stimuli;
- central modulation of pain stimuli, altering pain perception – most nociceptive pain is treated by locally (peripheral) acting analgesics.

### Controlling local tissue damage and release of inflammatory mediators

#### Pre-emptive analgesia

Pain can be controlled by anticipating the situations that are likely to cause it and then pre-emptively employing some strategy to reduce the impact of the stimulus or avoiding it entirely. This gives the practitioner more choices than might be initially obvious.

As mentioned previously, stimulating the aspects of the sensory nervous system that carry sensation centrally more quickly than pain fibres can cause a sensory blockade resulting in closing of the gate control mechanism. This may reduce the perception of pain, overriding the initial response to the noxious stimulus. An example outside the mouth is the instinctive rubbing of a body part that has been traumatised. This is often reflexive, but is also part of physical therapy such as massage. In the mouth, this technique might be used before local anaesthetic injection by rubbing, or putting pressure on the area of anticipated insertion of the needle immediately prior to the injection and immediately afterwards as well. Medications can also be employed in this manner such as topical local anaesthetic used before injection.

Local anaesthesia, or analgesia, will have the same effect, as it blocks the transmission of pain centrally, delaying or avoiding the onset of central sensitisation. Local anaesthesia is used to reduce the noxious stimuli of surgery under general anaesthesia and can reduce post-surgical pain scores. In a similar fashion, studies have shown that pre-emptive analgesics are more efficacious than placebo at reducing post-operative pain scores. This would suggest that analgesic control should start before the anticipated stimulus. It is still relatively unusual practice to employ this technique in clinical dentistry but is to be encouraged. Under local anaesthesia, due to blockade of the nerve stimulus during the damaging episode, central sensitisation will not take place until the reversal of the local anaesthetic effect. This provides a window of opportunity to prescribe analgesics to be taken before the return of sensation occurs. Anti-inflammatory medication given at this time, however, will not be so effective at controlling the release of inflammatory mediators, which will be initiated at the commencement of surgery.

### Reducing inflammation

The anticipated inflammatory response can be minimised in a variety of ways. Careful surgery with respect to the hard and soft tissues will reduce the inflammation. The use of cooled burs helps to reduce local damage to bone and gentle retraction of flaps can again reduce trauma and thus inflammation to the soft tissues.

Medications (such as steroids) can reduce post-operative inflammation, often employed after more traumatic surgical interventions.

An ice pack placed on the face may reduce the local inflammation and give symptomatic relief.

### Removal of the cause of inflammation

Simple though removal of the cause of inflammation is, this must not be avoided. Prompt attention to the cause of pain will limit the process and reduce possible analgesic requirements. Stop the trauma! - relieve dentures, reduce high restorations, encourage cessation of harmful habits such as nail biting.

Curing the infection, treating the periodontal problems and removing caries or necrotic pulps, if necessary, are vital steps in controlling pain stimuli. Extract involved teeth if required and institute incision and drainage. Reliance on analgesic medication alone to control dental pain will result in a poorer response.

## Blockade of nociceptive stimuli

The dental surgeon has an advantage in blocking nociceptive stimuli as local anaesthesia is paramount in achieving treatment goals. This blockade will certainly reduce central sensitisation but is designed to be temporary in nature. It may serve to help in achieving pre-emption of the pain but will reverse after a few hours. Longer acting agents (up to 12 hours) can be very helpful in some situations but are not always well tolerated by patients. The use of more permanent nerve-blocking strategies, for example cryotherapy, is usually reserved for chronic neuralgic pain.

## Central modulation of pain perception

Most of the agents used are either opioids or medications usually used to control epilepsy.

It must be made clear that these agents do not reduce the pain stimulus but alter the perception of pain centrally.

## Psychology of pain

Although pain experience helps to allow one to imagine another's pain, it is no indication of an individual's response to a particular stimulus. Perception of pain is extremely variable both within a population and also within an individual depending on the circumstances in which the experience takes place. The release of endorphins can help to reduce the perception of pain, although harnessing this effect in a clinical situation is more difficult.

That there is a strong emotional quality is not to be ignored and part of the management of pain requires the practitioner to understand and empathise with the experience as perceived by the patient. The use of behavioural techniques in the management of a patient in pain is extremely important and will tend to improve the outcome for many patients. The practitioner's role in this respect is to convince the patient that strategies can be employed to eliminate, reduce or control the symptoms.

## Placebo effect

The 'placebo effect' is another example of how the psychology of pain can alter outcomes. If the patient believes in the therapy, then it is more likely to work. Conversely, the efficacy of medication has to be contrasted with any possible placebo effect. Many drugs have failed to show a statistical advantage over placebo in controlled studies.

## Hypnosis

There is good evidence to support the efficacy of hypnosis in the control of acute and chronic pain and there is an active group of dental hypnotists who apply this in practice. The susceptible patient can accept the suggestion of pain control once in the hypnotic phase. In addition, hypnosis can be used to combat phobias that will increase patient anxiety and may sensitise subjects to pain stimuli. The effects of hypnosis are not eliminated by naloxone, an opioid antagonist, suggesting that these effects are not mediated by release of endorphins.

## Acupuncture

Acupuncture to interfere with pain pathways by stimulating specific points on the body that control these pathways has been practiced for centuries in Oriental medicine where it is common practice. The effect is coupled with a significant release of endorphins and the effect is inhibited by the action of naloxone.

## Psychogenic – non-organic pain

The practitioner should always make a careful diagnosis of the cause of pain and exhaust all possible pathological reasons for the presenting symptoms.

If no pathology is found to account for the patient's symptoms, the possibility of non-organic pain should be explored. On no account should patient insistence result in treatment of pathology-free dental units. This approach, if adopted can lead to serial extractions or root canal therapy with no resolution of the pain symptoms. Careful assessment and the use of reversible diagnostic therapies such as local anaesthetics and splints should be implemented to avoid irreversible dental damage:

- *Atypical facial pain*: Typically, this is pain associated with no identifiable dental pathology that can change in site, is poorly localised, does not necessarily respect anatomical boundaries and does not resolve with simple anti-inflammatory medication.
- *Burning mouth syndrome*: This affects the oral mucosa and is a 'dysaesthesia described as a burning sensation...' It may arise secondary to organic causes such as low Vitamin $B_{12}$ or folate, candidosis, or as an adverse drug reaction. Elimination of these possible causes should be undertaken before a final diagnosis is reached. Recent work has suggested that in some cases there may be more of an organic origin to this syndrome than was at first thought.

Control of these conditions can be extremely difficult and may prove to be impossible without the use of behavioural therapies. The management of patients with unremitting symptoms is often undertaken by a team of specialists with varying skills ranging from psychology to anaesthesia.

# Medication

## Steroids

Corticosteroids interrupt the synthesis of prostaglandins at the level of the action of phospholipase A on phospholipids from the cell membrane (Figure 8.3). Theoretically, this should be the most efficacious way of inhibiting the production of post-operative inflammatory mediators such as prostaglandins and bradykinin and thus pain. The use of steroids in this way is restricted by the possibility of adverse side effects with long courses and some questions over efficacy.

In other surgical specialties, their use is more widespread as part of a range of therapies to reduce analgesic requirements in the post-operative phase. In dentistry, however, most studies have not shown this and steroids are therefore mostly used in order to reduce the swelling that occurs due to the inflammatory response and consequent increase in vascular permeability. Patients may benefit from this effect alone as reduced swelling will give better post-operative function and a psychological boost. Their systemic use in dentistry is restricted to peri-operative prescription following more major surgery such as osteotomies or trauma. Topical steroids are sometimes used to control conditions such as lichen planus. Rarely, systemic steroids may be used.

## Locally acting analgesics (Table 8.4)

### Local anaesthetics

Local anaesthetics cause blockade of nerve impulses. This effect is due to stopping ionic transfer and consequent nerve depolarisation and conduction of stimuli. The effects are reversible and temporary. Commonly, lidocaine and adrenaline is used with a duration of action of up to 2.5 hours. Other allied preparations have prolonged activity. Bupivacaine has been used to control post-operative pain for up to 12 hours. Local anaesthetics can be extremely useful in controlling acute pain in the short term. They can also have diagnostic uses as non-organic pain is unlikely to be affected by local anaesthesia.

### Non-Steroidal Anti-Inflammatory Drugs

Non-steroidal anti-inflammatory drugs (NSAIDs) act to control prostaglandin synthesis at the level of thromboxane A2 (Figure 8.3). It is interesting that other inflammatory mediators will be little affected by these medications; thus, the development of the overall inflammatory response may not be affected. The principal medications used therapeutically are described in the succeeding sections.

### Aspirin

Aspirin, a derivative of salicylic acid, has been in use for many centuries as an analgesic and anti-inflammatory medication. It has a powerful effect on these mechanisms and still performs well against other newer NSAIDs in the control of post-operative pain. The side effects, which include gastric erosion, allergy, tinnitus and Reye's syndrome in younger patients, have limited its use to some degree but it is still widely prescribed. Its antiplatelet activity is used for prophylaxis at low doses against cardiovascular episodes. Therapeutic dosage is from 300 mg four times daily up to 600 mg four times daily. For cardiovascular prophylaxis, doses of 75 mg daily are effective.

### Ibuprofen

Ibuprofen is a potent analgesic and anti-inflammatory agent. It inhibits cyclooxygenase, thus interfering with prostaglandin synthesis. Since its introduction, ibuprofen has been very popular for relief of mild to moderate pain post-surgically. It is available in doses from 200–400 mg three times daily over-the-counter but can be prescribed under medical advice up to 800 mg three times daily. It has similar side effects to aspirin but is better tolerated.

### Diclofenac sodium

Diclofenac is a powerful anti-inflammatory analgesic used in the control of arthritis and post-surgical pain. It seems to act against cyclooxygenase in common with other NSAIDs but may also act against lipoxygenase, thus inhibiting the production of leukotrienes. Doses range from 25 mg to 50 mg three times daily.

**Table 8.4**  Peripherally acting analgesics.

| Classes | Action | Agents | Regimens | Cautions |
|---|---|---|---|---|
| Steroids | Inhibits eicosanoid production | Dexamethasone | 8 mg perioperatively | Long-term effects |
| NSAIDs | Inhibits prostaglandin synthesis, both cyclooxygenase-1 and 2 | Aspirin Ibuprofen Diclofenac | 600–1200 mg qds 200–400 mg tds 25–50 mg tds | Antiplatelet effect Gastric erosion |
| Cyclooxygenase-2 inhibitors | Selectively blocks cyclooxygenase-2 | Celecoxib | 200 mg once or twice daily | Cyclooxygenase inhibitors are associated with increased risks of MI (myocardial infarction) |
| | Peripheral anti-inflammatory effect – mild Central – antipyretic effect | Paracetamol | 500 mg–1 g qds | Overdosage causes liver damage |
| Local anaesthetics | Reversible nerve blockade | Lidocaine Bupivacaine | 2% ±epinephrine 0.25% ±epinephrine | Longer acting agents may be poorly tolerated |

### Specific cyclooxygenase inhibitors

A family of specific cyclooxygenase-2 inhibitors has been developed to try to focus on the inhibition of production of inflammatory mediators derived from prostaglandins without the gastrointestinal side effects of NSAIDs. Cyclooxygenase-2 is induced within inflamed tissues and thus can be specifically blocked to inhibit the development of the inflammatory response. This class of drug has shown some increased risk of development of cardiovascular disease due to sparing thromboxane-2 and inducing platelet aggregation due to inhibition of prostacyclin. Celecoxib appears to have a reduced risk of this side effect.

### Paracetamol

Paracetamol, or acetaminophen, is effective in controlling mild to moderate pain. Its action is thought to be by more than one mechanism alone. Firstly, it seems to be a specific cyclooxygenase-2 inhibitor and thus spares thromboxane A2 in prostaglandin synthesis. This means that it will act as an anti-inflammatory drug but it will have no anti-platelet activity. Secondly, paracetamol is thought to have some central activity by inhibiting production of prostaglandin E2, responsible for controlling temperature. Thus, paracetamol is a potent antipyretic. Thirdly, paracetamol inhibits uptake of endogenous cannabinoids by neurones, reducing activating of nociception.

Dosage ranges are from 250 mg four times daily to 1 g four times daily. Care must be taken not to overdose and patient's intake needs to monitored in order to avoid irreversible damage to the liver. Patients attending the dental emergency clinic who have been using over-the-counter paracetamol should be carefully questioned to elicit the actual amount they have taken. As little as 6 g per day over 48 hours could cause toxicity and if in doubt the patient should be sent for testing of paracetamol levels in the blood. As a matter of routine, when blood is sent for analysis of paracetamol levels, salicylate levels are ordered at the same time.

## Centrally acting analgesics (Table 8.5)

### Opioids

This group of substances affects endogenous receptors in the body and have been linked with a number of actions. They are potent modulators of the response to pain when they activate the endorphin system centrally but some studies have hinted at peripheral activity also, as opioid receptors have been demonstrated within many tissues, such as the periodontal ligament, but the activity of these receptors is less well defined. Pain thresholds seem to be raised by opioids as is tolerance of pain. The opioids also act in the gastrointestinal tract causing slowing and reduced force of contraction of the bowel, leading to constipation. Opioids cause sedation and respiratory depression. Opioids can occur as natural substances derived from poppies, principally morphine and codeine.

**Table 8.5** Centrally acting analgesics.

| Classes | Agents | Action | Regimens | Cautions |
|---|---|---|---|---|
| Opioids | Morphine<br>Tramadol<br>Codeine | Agonist at<br>opioid<br>receptors | 10 mg IM qds<br>50–100 mg qds<br>30–60 mg qds | Development<br>of tolerance<br>and addiction |
| GABA<br>derivatives | Gabapentin | May act on<br>GABA<br>receptors<br>Anti-epileptic | 300 mg<br>increasing to<br>maximum<br>1800 mg daily | Gradual<br>withdrawal due<br>to side effects |
| | Carbamazepine | Anti-epileptic<br>Stabilises<br>sodium<br>channels | 100 mg<br>increasing to<br>maximum 1600<br>mg daily | Hepatic and<br>renal damage<br>Leukopenia |
| | Amitriptyline | Tricyclic<br>antidepressant | 25–50 mg tds | Arrhythmias,<br>epilepsy,<br>hepatic<br>impairment |

IM, intramuscular; GABA, gamma-aminobutyric acid.

Overdose of opioids leads to respiratory depression. One sign of opioid use, particularly if the dosage is excessive, is the presence of the so-called pinpoint pupils, which refers to a state of marked pupil contraction.

### Morphine

Morphine was the first single alkaloid to be isolated from poppy extract in the early 1800s. It controls severe pain. It is used in the control of pain in the palliative care situation as well as acutely post-operatively, where its sedative effects and respiratory depression can cause management difficulties. The effect of morphine centrally makes any patient who has sustained a head injury more difficult to assess and care needs to be taken in its use in this environment. Tolerance to the effects of morphine can develop and also psychological addiction, well before physical addiction is established. It is unusual to consider morphine in post-operative pain control for dental causes but is frequently used after major maxillofacial or other operations. Doses of 5–10 mg should help to control pain in this period. As soon as possible, analgesic control should be established by other methods.

### Codeine

Codeine is also a naturally occurring alkaloid found in the poppy seed and is a very widely used opioid in the control of moderate pain. It is eventually metabolised to morphine but at much reduced amounts. Thus, it is less active than morphine but still causes reduced bowel motility, which is one of its therapeutic applications – control of diarrhoea. Physical dependence can occur as with morphine and overdosage can cause respiratory depression. Codeine is often combined with other medications, most frequently paracetamol, to improve the efficacy whilst keeping dosage down. Doses range from 10 mg to 50 mg.

### Tramadol

Tramadol is an analogue of codeine but does not metabolise to morphine. It is used to control moderate to severe pain, often of a chronic nature such as back pain. It has a place in controlling the pain of neuralgia but is little used in inflammatory pain of dental origin. Dosage is at 50 mg.

## Anti-epileptic drugs

### Gabapentin

Gabapentin was developed as an analogue of gamma-aminobutyric acid (GABA), a neurotransmitter, in order to mimic the chemical structure but it does not seem to act on the same receptors in the brain. It was originally designed as an antiepileptic medication but is now used to control neuropathic pain particularly in post-herpetic neuralgias.

### Carbamazepine

Carbamazepine is an anticonvulsant drug used in control of epilepsy and for the treatment of trigeminal neuralgia. Dosage starts at 100 mg twice daily and is increased incrementally to a maximum dose of 1600 mg per day until control of the pain is achieved. There are a number of side effects, the most significant of which is the potential development of aplastic anaemia. Regular blood counts should be performed whilst the patient is taking this medication.

## The ladder of analgesia

It is important in clinical practice that analgesics are prescribed in a methodical manner. To assist in this, it is useful to have a knowledge of the concept of the ladder of analgesia. In essence, this refers to a sequential approach to providing analgesia, matching the potency of the drug to the pain experienced by the patient. It commences with the use of paracetamol for mild pain and progresses with an addition of codeine, possibly supplemented with an NSAID such as ibuprofen in what might be termed moderate pain. In severe pain, paracetamol may be supplemented by a more potent opioid, possibly in addition to an NSAID.

## Avoiding problems in prescribing analgesics

All medications have the potential for harm. Awareness of these effects is important for the practitioner involved in their prescription. The first and vital step is to be aware of possible issues in the patient's medical history. Any liver disease, renal dysfunction or gastrointestinal ulceration needs to be considered, as well as other medication that the patient may be taking, which could potentiate the effect of the prescription or vice versa.

## Liver disease

The liver is the organ that is responsible for the metabolism of many drugs. If there is damage to the liver, this might potentiate the effect of the drug altering the safe dosage that may be prescribed. In addition, some analgesics such as paracetamol can cause liver damage and should be avoided or reached in dose if there is liver disease. Advice from the responsible physician should be sought. The British National Formulary should be consulted.

## Renal dysfunction

Prostaglandin activity is crucial to normal renal function. If this activity is reduced by use of NSAIDs, then further damage to the kidney may occur. NSAIDs should be avoided in renal dysfunction.

## Gastrointestinal ulceration

All NSAIDs may cause problems of gastric irritation or ulceration. This is particularly likely to occur if the prescription is long term. In fact, a short course for acute pain control is unlikely to produce any gastric erosion. However, in a patient who is already suffering from gastric ulceration, these drugs should be avoided. Anti-ulcer co-therapy in the form of antacids, histamine H2 blockers, proton pump inhibitors and prostaglandins may be taken to allow safe use of NSAIDs for the control of chronic pain, but their prescription lies outside the domain of the dental surgeon.

NSAIDs are widely prescribed by dental practitioners and it is important to be aware of other situations where their use may be restricted or contraindicated. A summary is given in Box 8.1.

## NSAID cautions

- Diabetic, elderly
- Vascular disease, asthma, renal failure

## NSAID contraindications

### Box 8.1    Cautions and contraindications in the prescription of NSAIDs

- Previous adverse reaction to NSAIDs including aspirin
- History or current peptic ulcer
- Current therapy with an NSAID
- Oral anticoagulant therapy
- Clotting problems
- Current deep vein thrombosis prophylaxis with low-molecular-weight heparin

## Cardiovascular risk

As stated previously, there appears to be an increased risk of developing cardiovascular disease in patients taking selective cyclooxygenase-2 inhibitors. Rofecoxib and valdecoxib have been withdrawn due to evidence supporting the increased risk of myocardial infarction and stroke in susceptible patients. Some risk may apply to non-selective cyclooxygenase inhibitors but there is no evidence to support this at present.

## Overdosage

Particular attention should be paid to ensuring that patients do not overdose on their analgesic medication. Overdosage is not particularly uncommon in a dental emergency clinic as some patients are attending as a last resort and have delayed presentation hoping that the problem will go away on its own and in the meantime have been taking excessive amounts of over-the-counter analgesics. The potential for harm is often underestimated. The practitioner should be aware of safe dosage levels and advise their patients accordingly. When prescribing, it should be ensured that the patient is not already prescribed another analgesic in the same class, which might increase the chance of inadvertent overdosage. One example of this is patients taking one of the codeine/paracetamol compound preparations, who also take paracetamol as the paracetamol content of the former is not recognised by the patient. If in any doubt about overdosage, the patient should be sent to accident and emergency for testing of blood analgesic levels.

## Summary

Diagnosis of the underlying cause of the pain will always be the cornerstone of effective prescribing. Once the diagnosis is known, there is a wide choice of peripherally acting analgesics that may be prescribed by the dentist to control pain of dental origin. However, paracetamol, either combined with codeine or alone, is a safe starting point, with Ibuprofen, as an adjunct to this, being effective in most circumstances. The so-called 'ladder of analgesia' should be used – gradually increasing drug potency depending on the response achieved.

Prescription will rely to some extent on experience and availability. Cost is also an issue and those medications easily available across the counter will be perfectly adequate to deal with the majority of situations that the practitioner will encounter.

Patients may also have preferences and what usually works for them will probably be a good choice.

## Further reading

British National Formulary (BNF). http://bnf.org.

Meechan J, Robb N, Seymour R, (1998) *Pain and Anxiety Control for the Conscious Dental Patient*. University Press, Oxford.

Ong C, Seymour R (2008) An evidence-based update of the use of analgesics in dentistry. *Periodontology 2000* **46**, 143-164.

# Chapter 9
# Management of the Special Needs Patient

## T. Nugent

## Introduction

In dentistry, patients with special needs may result in small alterations to standard practice or great challenges requiring hospital-based treatments. The special needs of patients with a disability of an intellectual, physical, sensory, emotional or behavioural nature may need a little more thought and understanding than those of the general population and these are discussed in this chapter.

### Definitions

In the area of special needs patients, definitions are constantly changing. The term 'learning disability' has the advantage of implying a permanent state of intellectual impairment, but disadvantages the less impaired with a potential stigma of being labelled 'disabled'. Many organisations would prefer no label to be used at all. People First, an international advocacy organisation, and Mencap have stated that 'learning difficulty' would be their preferred choice. In the United Kingdom, the government uses the term learning disability to describe specific problems of learning in children resulting from medical, emotional or communication impairment. The term intellectual disability is used in the United States and Australia. In healthcare and legislation, mental impairment may be used to identify whether the patient is able to consent for themselves (see later).

The general public tends to use many of these terms interchangeably. A summary of relevant terms is given in Table 9.1.

### People requiring individual care are commonplace

Approximately 985,000 people in England have a learning disability (2% of the population). The number of adults with learning disabilities is predicted

*Dental Emergencies*, First Edition. Edited by Mark Greenwood and Ian Corbett.
© 2012 Blackwell Publishing Ltd. Published 2012 by Blackwell Publishing Ltd.

**Table 9.1** Terminology used in patients with special needs.

| Term | Definition |
| --- | --- |
| Impairment | An injury, illness, or congenital condition that causes or is likely to cause a long-term effect on appearance and/or limitation of function of the individual. |
| Disability | The loss or limitation of opportunities to take part in society on an equal level with others due to social and environmental barriers. |
| Handicap | Social experience as a result of the impairment or disability. |
| Special needs | An inclusive term for people who do not fit perfectly into standard practice. |
| Learning disability | (1) Covers many different intellectual disabilities. Inferring a person's capacity to learn is affected and that they may not learn things as quickly as other people.<br>(2) 'A state of arrested or incomplete development of mind, with significant impairment of intellectual functioning' and 'significant impairment of adaptive/social functioning' (World Health Organisation). |
| Learning difficulty | Infers specific problems with learning in children that might arise as a result of a number of different things, e.g. medical problems, emotional problems, language impairments, etc. (Warnock Committee). |
| Intellectual disability | Characterised both by a significantly below-average score on a test of mental ability or intelligence and by limitations in the ability to function in areas of daily life, such as communication, self-care, and getting along in social situations and school activities. Intellectual disability is sometimes referred to as a cognitive disability or mental retardation, but the latter has pejorative connotations in popular discourse. |
| Special needs | A person who has a disability of an intellectual, physical, sensory, emotional or behavioural nature, has a learning disability or has exceptional gifts or talents (used in United States). |
| Mental impairment | A disorder characterised by the display of an intellectual defect, as manifested by diminished cognitive, interpersonal, social and vocational effectiveness and quantitatively evaluated by psychological examination and assessment. Used in legal matters Mental Health Act, 1983. |

to increase by 11% between 2001 and 2021, raising the number of people in England aged 15 years and above with learning disabilities to more than a million by 2021.

The number of adults with learning disabilities aged more than 60 years is predicted to increase by 36% between 2001 and 2021, according to the Institute for Health Research at Lancaster University.

It is estimated that approximately 3 per 1000 people in the United Kingdom community have what is considered a severe learning disability, and 25 per

1000 have a mild to moderate learning disability. These figures are comparable to other westernised societies.

## Commonly seen conditions

People with learning disabilities are 2.5 times more likely to have health problems than other people, according to the Disability Rights Commission. Learning disabilities may be congenital or acquired.

Down syndrome is the most common condition associated with learning difficulties, accounting for 60,000 people in the United Kingdom, and 750 births per annum. There is a wide spectrum of intellect within this syndrome, ranging from mild to severe impairment. With the increasing numbers of aging mothers, the incidence of Down syndrome is rising, as is life expectancy.

Patients with Down syndrome tend to understand more than their level of verbal communication might suggest. If there is a chaperone, they will hopefully help establish the best method and level of communication. Complicating factors such as a higher association with dementia and more specifically Alzheimer's disease from the age of 40 onwards may hamper communication further.

Studies have not shown a higher caries prevalence in people with Down syndrome, but the incidence of poor oral hygiene and consequent periodontal disease is high. Plaque scores have been recorded as being poor in 80% of people with the disease. It should not be a surprise to have a Down syndrome patient attend as an emergency with acute necrotising ulcerative gingivitis or a periodontal abscess.

Dementia, the most common form being Alzheimer's disease, has a generalised increased risk for aging people with learning difficulties. Prevalence in this group is four times that of the general population. Self-care and dexterity may see a decline if adequate intervention is not provided. These patients may not present until in pain.

One in five people with epilepsy have learning difficulties, although neither condition causes the other. The incidence of epilepsy associated with learning difficulties is at least ten times higher than the general population and is also associated with social deprivation. Epilepsy is the most common childhood neurological disorder and has been associated with increased risk of dental trauma. The most common type of seizure experienced, if the patient has concordant learning difficulties, is the tonic-clonic type. This in turn is associated with higher risk of trauma.

Children with epilepsy have been found to have higher plaque scores than the general public but not necessarily higher caries rates. This would tend to suggest that they have equal risk of presenting with irreversible pulpitis due to caries as the rest of the general public but a higher risk of acute periodontal conditions.

Mental health disorders differ from learning difficulties as they tend to have an adult onset, may be temporary and do have medical and other treatments available. One in four of the general population will have a mental health issue at some point in their lifetime, usually transiently. These conditions tend to be more prevalent in people with learning disabilities, increasing to up to 40%. All of these conditions may make dental treatment more challenging and result in more people with special needs requiring emergency treatment due to limited preventative dental treatment.

As the majority of people with known learning disability live in the community, it is not rare to see people with learning disabilities in general dental practices or at emergency dental clinics. The Disability Discrimination Acts 1995 and 2005 have made discrimination illegal and the General Dental Council encourages positive attitudes towards no discrimination.

The history can be difficult in these patients and pain tolerance higher. Patients with greater special needs will require longer appointments; this clearly has a direct bearing on the ability to carry out a full assessment.

## Assessment

Patients with greater special needs will require longer appointments.

Prior to the patient coming through to the surgery preferably, if possible, a written medical history form should be completed and examined. This is useful preparation, as it facilitates research if the patient attends with a rare condition. Alternatively, practitioners may need to contact a GP or hospital consultant for advice. Often, patients attend with a member of the care team who is not familiar with the patient and contact with the matron/manager of the care home for further information about the patient is essential. Only reputable websites should be used for information gathering. Understanding of the patient's situation will go a long way to gaining the trust of both patient and chaperone.

If the patient is wheelchair bound, taking a few minutes to check the path to the surgery or dental chair is clear will also give a more prepared, professional feel to the appointment. Any special equipment for transfer or comfort (such as a pillow) should be at hand. The surgery should be kept peaceful with minimal distractions. Only the necessary staff should be present and efforts should be made to avoid people coming in and interrupting the consultation or treatment session.

It is important to make a good impression with any patient and often in emergency appointments the practitioner may not know the patient. Always greet the patient first and the chaperone second. It should never be assumed that because someone is in a wheelchair or has a carer that they cannot comprehend or communicate. Disease processes such as multiple sclerosis will physically incapacitate a patient before any intellectual impairment occurs, if indeed such impairment happens at all.

Suggestions for effective communication with someone with a learning disability include maintaining eye contact, smiling and using a normal voice, speaking clearly using simple language. The practitioner should always start by identifying themselves and addressing the patient by name to establish communication. Practitioners should avoid overloading the patient with questions; for example, by asking only one pertinent question at a time and waiting for a response before moving on. If the patient has not heard clearly, the question should be repeated exactly. If the patient has not understood, simplify the question. When giving instructions, pace and repeat them. Break down treatment into stages to simplify what is being requested of the patient. Suggest breaks during treatment.

For hearing impaired patients, practitioners must always talk face-to-face to allow lip reading and if possible request a professional signing interpreter. Unfortunately, having an interpreter attend at short notice may be difficult. Ask if a relative or friend who signs can attend. If there is nobody available, it may be necessary to write questions and answers down. To establish some form of communication and trust, the practitioner could try basic signing. There are many websites that will explain the basic symbols and alphabet. Even if there is limited verbal communication, 'show tell do' is an effective method of visual communication.

The visually impaired patient should always be approached from the front. Very few people who are registered blind have no sight at all; perception and shadows are usually recognised. The patient should only be touched with their permission and visually impaired patients may be hypersensitive to touch. When discussing treatment, descriptive terms should be used about the other remaining senses, such as how something will taste, smell, feel and sound.

## Medical history in the patient with special needs

It is worth going through the patient's medical history with them and if present, their chaperone. Often, people with specific conditions, or their relatives will know their condition in depth.

Patients and chaperones may not always comprehend what is meant by the question posed and may not include very obvious facts, as living with an impairment everyday may not feel to them like a disability. For example, patients with limited manual dexterity may not be fully aware of its extent. There are many patients that are completely unaware of having a learning disability, only 20% of adults with learning disabilities are known to learning disability services. It is important for informed consent to be obtained that it is established that the patient can comprehend.

Medical histories can be particularly long and complex in this patient group. There are many good websites such as emedicine.medscape.com/ and www.gpnotebook.co.uk/ for basic conditions, as well as charity-based sites for specific rare conditions. The British National Formulary online (bnf.org/bnf/) is an excellent up-to-date resource for therapeutic treatments. The medical emergencies box and oxygen should be nearby as a matter of routine for all patients. The management of medical emergencies is discussed in detail in Chapter 11.

## History – other aspects

Discussion about the patient's symptoms, previous dental treatments, anxieties and social history should be carried out. Practitioners should resist the temptation to be judgmental about the care the patient may be receiving, but if there are concerns that the patient is being neglected or not receiving the level of care they need, this may be discussed further with the patient, their general medical practitioner or the department in the appropriate trust that deals with vulnerable adults.

Do not forget that this group of patients may be dentally phobic as well as having learning disabilities.

## Informed consent

In adult patients, the time speaking to both patient and carer enables an informed decision to be made about the patient's mental capacity. The area of consent is also discussed in Chapter 2. If the practitioner feels the adult patient does not satisfy the two-stage test (Box 9.1) for capacity, then it must be established if there are any advance directives or power of attorney required, or if there is any fluctuation in their capacity to understand and if a delay to treatment is appropriate.

---

**Box 9.1   Assessment of capacity, two-stage test**

(1) Does the patient have an impairment of brain or mental function?
(2) Does this impairment result in a disability that does not allow them to make a specific decision?

---

The Mental Capacity Act 2005, states that nobody other than the patient can give consent for another adult. If that person lacks capacity, then one must act in their best interests when providing treatment. The only caveat to this is if the patient has made advance directives or appointed a Lasting Power of Attorney to another person.

A patient consenting for themselves is always best. If it is thought that they have fluctuating mental capacity with relapsing and remitting disease, such as in the early stages of dementia, then if treatment is deemed non-urgent, delaying it until another appointment when consent may be gained is preferential. Where treatment is imperative and it is felt that the patient cannot consent, discussion with the family should take place with regard to what the practitioner feels is in the patient's best interests and with their agreement, proceed. If the family does not agree, then non-urgent treatment can be overseen and mediated with an Independent Mental Capacity Advocate, and if this is still in debate, via a court of law. For urgent treatment, the practitioner is expected by law to act in the best interests of the patient. It may be wise to get a second opinion from a colleague, if they are available, and to contact a Dental Defence society, if concerned.

For an examination, as with any other patient, implied consent with the patient sitting and opening the mouth is adequate. For treatment, written consent is preferred and documentation of the level of capacity of the patient should be ensured.

## Examination

If the patient is able-bodied and not anxious, examination can be carried out in the dental chair. For those patients with hyperactivity disorders, such as attention deficit hyperactivity disorder, examination should be carried out effectively but quickly. The environment should be simple – no instruments left out, suction switched off, radio switched off. The use of intended distraction may be helpful in an otherwise simplified environment. Working as a team in this circumstance is essential, as it will allow options to be discussed with parents or carers whilst the nurse distracts and prevents the patient from harming themselves. If the patient is on sedatives, scheduling the appointment when they are most subdued will sometimes be very helpful.

If the patient is in a wheelchair, it should be established whether safe transfer to the chair is required and possible without risking damage to the patient, the clinician or the staff. If the clinic has suitable transfer equipment, for example a banana slide board or hoist and staff are trained in manual handling, then with the help of the carer or family, the patient can be transferred safely. If not, treatment in the wheelchair is the next best option. Ideally, for the patient a headrest is best but this is not always possible.

### Special investigations

Depending on the special needs of the patient, radiographs and vitality, testing may or may not be possible. Segmental panoramic radiographs may be preferred to intra-oral views in patients with prominent gag reflexes. If a radiograph is not possible but would have usually been part of the treatment plan, a note should be made that one has not been taken and why.

## Factors to consider in treatment

Treatment plans for patients with learning disabilities should be made on an individual basis with a large measure of common sense being applied. The best interests of the patient are always the treatment of choice, but where the ideal treatment is not possible, compromised treatment plans may have to be made in the short term. For some patients, referral to tertiary care for sedation or general anaesthetic may be required. It is not possible to summarise how to treat hundreds of thousands of people in one chapter, so included are some general principles and a few techniques specific to the more common conditions.

Patient and family expectations must be taken into account when deciding on a treatment plan. Even if a patient has severe learning disabilities, it does not mean that they do not deserve to keep a beautiful smile. Patients should not be 'written off' because their chaperone has a lack of interest in them and their care.

Practical general advice includes the use of rubber dam where there is a risk of aspiration, but only if the patient can breathe through their nose and has sufficient compliance. Good aspiration is essential as is the use of finger rests to cope with sudden or rhythmic movements.

Care when using local anaesthetic or rotary equipment is essential as sudden movements can cause damage and needlestick injury. Clearly, patients should be kept as relaxed as possible. If consent has been achieved and the patient is happy, gentle stabilisation of their head by the chaperone may be carried out to assist in preventing harm. A mirror should be used for retraction, if possible.

If the best treatment for that patient is dental extraction under local anaesthetic, then that is the treatment that should be attempted. However, if that patient will not allow extraction without general anaesthetic but will allow the practitioner to temporise the tooth, then that would be the compromised treatment of choice until definitive care can be elicited. More complex treatment options, for example molar endodontics, may be appropriate in some cases but the overall patient context should always be borne in mind.

The incidence of incisal trauma is higher in patients with poorly controlled epilepsy (see Chapter 7). Prevention using upper and lower soft splints (especially over the upper teeth) is encouraged. Splints must be very well fitting, with good gingival coverage and may reduce both hard and soft tissue trauma. Unfortunately, even in patients who wear the splints conscientiously, seizures can occur at meal times when the splint may not be being worn. The principles of trauma management are essentially the same. In patients where there is no compliance for restoration, extraction may need to be considered with or without the use of general anaesthetic. Tertiary referral services vary regionally and it is important to establish local availability.

In patients with conditions that might result in poor facial neurological control, such as multiple sclerosis (MS), who will have limited ability to tolerate dentures in the long term, concerted efforts should be made to retain the natural dentition for as long as possible. In the early stages of MS, movements will be manageable and are not as pronounced in the maxilla, making treatment feasible. Finger rests in the same arch can be helpful as the dental surgeon may move with the patient. Keeping the patient relaxed is very important. Often, the harder the patient tries to keep still, the more they move, so relaxation and gentle hypnosis may be useful techniques. As the disease progresses, restoration may not be possible and extraction more likely.

In patients with dementia, the use of a blanket or soft toy may comfort them during treatment. Fatigue should be prevented in elderly confused patients by allowing periods of rest.

## Signs of abuse

Abuse is defined as any act, or failure to act, which results in a significant breach of a vulnerable person's human rights, civil liberties, bodily integrity, dignity or well-being. This includes exploitative sexual relationships and financial transactions to which the person has not, or cannot, validly consent.

Unfortunately, people with learning disabilities do suffer neglect and abuse on occasion. Such neglect is not, of course, confined to patients with special needs, it should be remembered as a possibility in any patient group where suspicions are raised. Neglect can be obvious but also unintentional. After discussion with the patient, referral to their general medical practitioner or social services for additional support may help to rectify the situation and create a more helpful care plan for that individual. Where neglect is intentional, the dental professional may be the only member of the healthcare team to see the patient. It is essential to refer the patient on and not rely or assume that others know about the situation.

Signs of sexual and mental abuse can be similar to those experienced by others who do not have learning disabilities but may be masked by already abnormal behaviour or a lack of emotional expression. If there is a frenal tear or palatal bruising, the method of injury should be questioned. For children, referral is through the regular child protection pathway. For adults, referral is through the vulnerable adults pathway.

Box 9.2 constitutes ten pointers that should be considered when suspicions of abuse arise. None of them is pathognomonic on its own, neither does the absence of any of them preclude the diagnosis of abuse.

---

### Box 9.2   Factors to consider if patient abuse is suspected

(1) Could the injury have been caused accidentally and if so how?

(2) Does the explanation for the injury fit the age and the clinical findings?

(3) If the explanation of the cause is consistent with the injury, is this itself within normally acceptable limits of behaviour.

(4) Has there been a delay in seeking medical help? Are there good reasons for this?

(5) Is the story of the 'accident' vague, lacking in detail, and does it vary with each telling and from person to person?

(6) The relationship between parent or carer and child patient.

(7) The patient's reaction to other people and any medical/dental examination.

(8) The general demeanour of the patient.

(9) Any comments made by the patient and/or parent/carer that gives cause for concern about the patient's lifestyle or upbringing.

(10) History of a previous injury.

## Record keeping

As with all patients, practitioners must keep accurate written records of examinations, medical histories and treatments. Written notes will be as standard but with additional information about patient capacity and if this was considered to be impaired, how was that decided? If the patient had a fluctuating capacity, whether it was felt the practitioner could wait to treat a non-urgent condition with informed consent or if it was felt the practitioner had to act in the patient's best interests on that day should be recorded. Names of family members involved in the decision-making process should also be recorded.

If it was felt that the treatment plan was compromised because of the patient's ability to cooperate, then the reasoning behind this should be recorded. Further steps taken to rectify the dental emergency, for example referral to tertiary care for extraction under general anaesthetic, should be included.

## Aftercare

Both patient and chaperone should have any warnings, advice and follow-up treatment required explained to them. The patient must have access to follow-up care, either with a general dental practitioner or in community or hospital based services. Any urgent referrals should be made. Leaflets on treatment should be made available to patients, including those in Braille or with larger writing for partially sighted individuals.

## Conclusion

Patients with special needs require particularly bespoke treatment planning, sometimes requiring a great deal of ingenuity. The ideal is to prevent the patient from needing emergency treatment as far as possible, through education regarding diet, sugar-free medication, good oral hygiene, the use of fluoride and introducing gum shields in patients prone to seizures. The emergency patient should be given a further point of reference whether that be in the community, hospital or general dental service.

# Chapter 10
# Making a Referral

## I.P. Corbett and J. Greenley

## Introduction

A referral is essentially a request for assistance regarding a patient, from an appropriate colleague. This may be a referral from primary care to secondary care or occasionally between clinicians in secondary care. Common principles apply to both. The referring practitioner may require a second opinion, or in many cases, the referral may also request that management of a patient be undertaken. Such a referral requires the transfer of information between the referring dental surgeon and, in many cases, a specialist, and may take a verbal, electronic or written form. Often, the referral may be an elective process following discussion between the patient and clinician regarding treatment options. However, on other occasions, the referral may require the prompt attention of a specialist to deal with an urgent concern raised by the patient or clinician. In order to facilitate the efficient referral of a patient, a few simple principles should be followed and these are discussed later.

## When to refer

According to the General Dental Council's 'Standards for Dental Professionals', 2009, registered dentists are expected to:

1.3 Work within your knowledge, professional competence and physical abilities. Refer patients for a second opinion and for further advice when it is necessary, or if the patient asks. Refer patients for further treatment when it is necessary to do so.

As such, the need for referral may be that the situation lies outside:

- the knowledge;
- the skill;

*Dental Emergencies*, First Edition. Edited by Mark Greenwood and Ian Corbett.
© 2012 Blackwell Publishing Ltd. Published 2012 by Blackwell Publishing Ltd.

159

- the experience; or
- the facilities available to the referring dentist.

Knowledge and skills may change with time as experience is gained, or postgraduate training is undertaken. Conditions that may be referred in the early stages of a clinician's career may be something that can be managed confidently later. Therefore, it is important that practitioners recognise their own level of competence. When deciding not to refer, then the clinician must be certain that they can manage the situation with the patient's safety and best interests in mind.

In a profession in which time and monetary issues are frequently influences on treatment, it must be considered whether it is acceptable or indeed ethical to refer a patient for the management of a complaint that the referring dentist is capable of managing in every other respect. Referral of such cases increases the workload of the person or department receiving the referral and will inevitably lead to delays in managing patients that require more urgent or specialist care.

## How to refer

The most common form a referral takes is that of a letter. Many attempts have been made to produce standard pro forma letters to simplify the process of referral. Standard letters are also considered by some to improve the information, which is provided by prompting the referrer for information. However, a written letter allows flexibility in the approach and a full description of a patient's condition. The disadvantage of any written medium is ensuring that it reaches its destination in a timely manner, or indeed that it reaches its destination at all. Where an urgent referral is required, letters may be faxed. Faxing a letter may produce a record that the letter was sent, although not that it was received. In many cases, an identical letter is faxed and a copy also sent by mail. Where this is the case, it is important to mark the posted letter as a copy, in order that a duplicate appointment is not arranged, as it may be difficult to identify and match duplicate letters. Emergency referrals may also be made by telephone call. It is important to keep a record of the telephone conversation, and best practice is to follow this up with a letter. The letter should refer to the telephone conversation and provide the appropriate details expected in any referral. The use of electronic mail or online referral of patients has yet to become common practice, but many centres are now developing this service.

When a referral is made, it is important to retain a copy of correspondence in the patient's records for medico-legal reasons. It may also be good practice or, depending on local policy, necessary to send a copy of the correspondence to the patient.

Patient confidentiality should be maintained at all times. Letters and faxes should be marked as confidential, as by their very nature they contain patient identifiable data and sensitive clinical information.

## Where to refer

Careful consideration should be made with regard to where, and whom to refer a patient. Secondary care and specialist services are generally provided by district general hospitals and teaching hospitals. The community dental service may also accept referrals. Practitioners should consider what service the patient requires. In some cases, more than one service may be necessary. Where a single referral letter containing multiple unrelated requests is sent, this may delay treatment. The department receiving the referral initially may deal with the relevant issue to completion before returning the patient to the referrer with remaining issues unresolved. Referring for unrelated items is usually best done by individual letters to each appropriate department.

Most receiving units will 'triage' referral letters. The information contained within each letter is examined to determine the nature of the referral and the degree of urgency. The referral may then be 'graded', for example as urgent or routine and placed on an appropriate waiting list. Such triage ensures that, where sufficient detail is provided, potentially urgent issues are identified and treated as such. Although referral may be made to a named consultant, in order to minimise waiting times, the patient may be seen by another appropriate consultant. Similarly, specialists within a department may have different sub-specialty interests and referrals may be redirected to the most appropriate person.

If the practitioner is unsure as to whom to refer, it may be acceptable to refer to 'the consultant' in the most relevant department, with redirection by that person on receipt. This again may delay the patient being seen, and it may be better practice to contact the referral centre or department by phone for advice. This will ensure that the correct person receives the referral promptly.

## The referral letter

The minimum data that a referral letter must include is summarised in Box 10.1 and an example of a 'good' referral letter is given in Figure 10.1.

> ### Box 10.1   Minimum data to be included in the letter of referral
>
> - Referring dentist's name, address and a telephone number
> - The patient's name, date of birth, address and telephone number
> - An indication of the urgency of the referral
> - The presenting complaint
> - History of the presenting complaint
> - Clinical findings
> - Relevant medical history
> - Whether an opinion or management is sought

**Hospital NHS Trust (Dental Hospital)**
Tel No: 0123 456789 **Letter of referral**     Fax No: 0123 567890

| | | |
|---|---|---|
| ☐ Conservation | ☐ Child Dental | **X** Oral Surgery |
| ☐ Orthodontics | ☐ Radiology | ☐ Sedation |
| ☐ Periodontics | ☐ Oral Medicine | ☐ P rosthodontic |

Title: *Mr*                                    Sex:   M /~~F~~

Surname:     *Smith*                   First Name:   *John*

Surname at Birth:     *N/A*       Middle name: *Albert*

Address:     *1 The Street, City*       Date of Birth: *6 June 66*

Postcode:     *AB1 2CD*               NHS Number: *123-456-7890*

Telephone     Home: *0123 567 8910*     Mobile:     *0789 101112*

                    Work: *01223 456 7890*

Ambulance Patient:   ~~Y~~ / N

**Registered GDP**                          **Registered GMP**

Name: *Dr A.N Other*                Name: *Dr G Practice*

Address: *The Dental Practice, City*     Address: *The Surgery, City*

Postcode: *AB2 3EF*                 Postcode: *AB3 4GH*

Telephone No: *345 6789*           Telephone No: *456 7890*

Dear Professor Smith,

I am writing to refer the above named patient for assessment and subsequent treatment of a grossly carious 46, the tooth is being unrestorable. The 46 has been dressed and the patient is currently asymptomatic, as such an urgent appointment is not required.

Mr Smith had a laryngeal cancer treated in City General Hospital, December 2009, managed with surgery and subsequent radiotherapy. No other medical problems were noted, the patient currently taking no medication. Mr Smith smokes 20 cigarettes per day and is a non-drinker.

I enclose a recent periapical radiograph and would be grateful for its return on completion of treatment.

Signed:         *A.N Other*         Print Name:   A.N. Other     Date:   1 January 11

Please return to: Records Department, Dental Hospital, Hospital NHS Trust, City, AB1 2CD.

**Figure 10.1**   An example of a 'good' referral letter that contains all the salient information that the receiver needs to know.

In addition to those factors listed in Box 10.1, if the patient has been referred in the past, reference numbers or patient identifier numbers of the receiving centre should also be clearly stated as these will facilitate recall of existing notes and correspondence, greatly assisting in the management of the patient.

Other than the essential demographic data required to contact the patient, the nature of the problem is the next most important information. This should follow the order of a simple patient assessment. Where appropriate, the patient's presenting complaint and history of the complaint should be given, along with the treatment history subsequent to presentation. Clinical findings should be summarised as follows:

- Accurate description of site size and nature of lesion(s)
- A brief report of radiographic findings
- Results of other investigations

If the referral concerns a soft tissue lesion, for example an oral mucosal white patch, it is important to describe the lesion as accurately as possible. Details such as the size, shape, colour, homogenicity, and so forth of the lesion are important. This may be supplemented by an intra-oral clinical photograph, simple diagram or 'mouth map'.

Including the results of any investigations, which may have been performed in or with the referral letter, may prevent duplication of effort. This is particularly true of radiographs. Including radiographs with the referral will prevent unnecessary further exposure to radiation. Where a radiograph is mentioned in a letter, or the patient reports having had a radiograph taken that may aid diagnosis or treatment, the receiving practitioner has a duty to request the radiograph, which will inevitably delay the patient's management. Standard radiograph films are acceptable, as are digital images, generally provided on disk with the necessary viewing software as appropriate. Where images are stored digitally for transport, this should be in line with local confidentiality regulations, for example the use of encryption, or via secure e-mail servers. Printouts of digital images should be provided on high-quality photographic paper, as plain paper copies are rarely of diagnostic quality and are not defensible for use medico-legally. Where previous images are not of diagnostic quality, this should be stated in the letter.

It is good practice to indicate at the bottom of the referral letter what items are included. This serves as a reminder to place the item in the envelope so that these may be identified and not misplaced on receipt. A gentle reminder to return radiographs to the practitioner following their use will not bring offence. Often, in the dental emergency clinic, patients will not have had radiographs taken. It is still important to check with the patient as duplication should be avoided wherever possible.

A summary of the patient's medical history, especially any history that may be relevant to the current complaint is essential. This may take the form of a copy of the practice's recent medical history form. Patients frequently forget the names of their current medication and therefore a list of medications that that practitioner is aware that the patient may be taking can be useful.

Other information that will assist in the referral procedure may relate to social history or patient needs. Identifying patients who require ambulance transport to appointments will allow appropriate appointment times to be given and will prevent missed appointments. Where patients have mobility issues, an indication of the need for hoists or lifts will allow the necessary equipment to be available at the patient's appointment. The need for interpreting services, indicating language and dialect where appropriate, should be clearly stated.

Finally, an indication of what the practitioner would like the person to whom referral is made to do will assist in subsequent treatment planning. For example, rather than:

*'I would be most grateful if you could arrange to see Joe Bloggs'*

it may be more useful to state:

*'I am writing to refer the above named patient for assessment and subsequent treatment of. . . .'*

or

*'I would be most grateful for an opinion regarding . . . I am happy to provide the necessary treatment'.*

An indication of the extent to which the practitioner is willing or able to participate in the relevant treatment is helpful.

## Urgency

An indication of the urgency of a referral should be included in the referral letter. This should be appropriate to the specific condition of the patient. Where the referrer can provide acute management of a problem, this should be undertaken prior to referral, for example accessing and dressing a tooth with irreversible pulpitis prior to an endodontic referral. The referrer should also continue to provide necessary care of the patient prior to the referral appointment and continue to manage the oral of health of the patient as appropriate throughout the consultation period.

The most urgent referrals are those of suspected cancers, and these are specifically dealt with as discussed later.

Other urgent referrals include patients with following problems:

- Possible airway risk:
  - Complaining of difficulty swallowing or speaking
- Patients who are systemically unwell:
  - Pyrexia, fever, rigors, tachycardia, tachypnoea

Such patients should be referred to a maxillofacial surgery unit or emergency department by telephone and, where necessary, by ambulance.

Abscesses, failed extractions, oro-antral communications and similar conditions that can be given acute management in primary care do not generally require an urgent referral. These patients should be managed appropriately and can then be referred on an elective basis.

## Cancer referrals

Cancer referral guidelines were produced by the Department of Health in March 2000 to support the government's initiative that all patients with a suspected cancer should be seen within 2 weeks. The guideline was subsequently updated by the National Institute for Health and Clinical Excellence in June 2005.

The so-called 2-week rule should be used when a patient presents with features typical of a head and neck cancer, or when there are unusual symptoms or symptoms that fail to resolve as expected where cancer may be a possibility.

Diagnosis of a cancer on clinical presentation alone may not be possible and diagnosis generally requires special investigations. Where there is a suspicion of a cancer, referral to a specialist should not be delayed by carrying out further investigations in primary care or a dental emergency clinic (Table 10.1). Where there is uncertainty whether a referral is required, most specialists will be happy to discuss and advise via a telephone contact. However, if in doubt, refer.

When referring a patient with a suspected cancer, a decision must be made about what information to give to the patient. Patients have an ethical right to know the nature of and the reasons for the referral. When suspicions are left unspoken, the patient will often assume that the diagnosis is cancer, and an opportunity to reassure the patient and allay fears will have been missed. Two weeks is a long time to endure fears with no means of support. The referrer should be willing and able to give patients information on the possible diagnosis and patients are often reassured that referral and investigations are to exclude the suspicion of cancer. Information given to the patient should generally include the items summarised in Box 10.2.

---

**Box 10.2   Information to be given to a patient attending with a suspected oral malignancy**

- Why the referral is being made?
- Where the patient is being referred to?
- How long they should expect to wait for the appointment?
- What to expect at the referral appointment?
- That further investigations are often required.
- That they may wish to be accompanied at the appointment.

---

Patients may need continuing support during this time and it is good practice to give the opportunity to contact or attend the practice or department for further information or advice prior to their referral appointment. Most patients will not make use of such an invitation, but it is reassuring to have a point of contact. Similarly, patients may often wish to discuss or clarify outcomes following the referral appointment and this should be facilitated.

**Table 10.1** Referral guidelines for mouth cancer and other oral mucosal conditions, based on recommendations produced by Cancer Research (United Kingdom).

| Type of referral | Example | Refer to |
|---|---|---|
| Urgent (within 2 wk) NICE, 2005 | • Unexplained oral ulceration or mass persisting for more than 3 wk<br>• Unexplained red, or red and white patches that are painful, swollen or bleeding<br><br>If patches are not painful, swollen or bleeding, referral can be made non-urgently. | The local oral and maxillofacial surgery, ENT or plastic surgery unit. |
| | • Unexplained one-sided pain in the head and neck area for more than 4 wk, associated with ear ache, but with a normal otoscopy<br>• Unexplained recent lump in the neck, or a previously undiagnosed lump that has changed over a period of 3–6 wk<br>• Unexplained persistent sore or painful throat<br>• Signs and symptoms in the oral cavity persisting for more than 6 wk that cannot be definitively diagnosed as a benign lesion<br>• Unexplained tooth mobility persisting for more than 3 wk that cannot be attributed to a dental cause | Referrals can be done by telephone or fax, or by filing out a 2WW (2 wk wait) referral form, depending on arrangements with local specialist units. |
| | Hoarseness persisting for more than 3 weeks, especially in smokers aged more than 50 yr, and heavy drinkers. | A chest X-ray. If positive, refer urgently to a team specialising in lung cancer. If negative, refer urgently to a team specialising in head and neck cancer. |
| Prompt | • Lichen planus. Patients with confirmed oral lichen planus should be monitored for oral cancer as part of a routine dental examination<br>• White patches with no redness or ulceration<br>• Chronic hyperplastic/ pseudomembranous candidosis<br>• Oral sub-mucous fibrosis<br>• Painful traumatic ulcers<br>• Recent unilateral salivary gland swellings<br>• Mucositis | A specialist unit by the normal route (usually, a written referral). If you have doubts about the urgency of a lesion, phone the local maxillofacial surgery, oral medicine, oral surgery or plastic surgery unit to consult a specialist. |

*(Continued)*

**Table 10.1** (*Continued*).

| Type of referral | Example | Refer to |
| --- | --- | --- |
| Non-urgent | • Polyps<br>• Mucoceles<br>• Pyogenic granulomas<br>• Areas of lichenoid reactions<br>• Amalgam tattoos<br>• Recurrent oral ulcers | As in prompt |

NICE, National Institute for Health and Clinical Excellence; ENT, ear nose tongue.

Cancer referrals should be clearly marked as such, for example '2-week rule' or 'suspected cancer'. Referrals from dental or medical practitioners should be made by fax and a copy sent by post, marked as such. A telephone call to confirm receipt is good practice. When received, the specialist has 2 weeks from the date of referral in which to see the patient. Inevitably, some patients may be unable to attend appointments offered and every effort will be made to accommodate the patient at the earliest opportunity. Receiving centres/departments have defined protocols and monitored pathways with specific timelines for the management of such patients. The specialist should keep the referrer informed of the outcome of appointments and where appropriate also inform the patient's general medical practitioner.

It is important that the 2-week rule is not abused. Conditions other than suspected cancers should not be referred in this manner. An example of a letter of referral for a patient with suspected cancer being referred under the 2-week rule is shown in Figure 10.2.

## Copies of the referral letter

As previously mentioned, there are usually local policies and procedures in place when considering to whom a copy of a referral should be sent. Hence, it is important to be aware of any pre-existing policies and comply with these whilst working in any given institution.

Potential recipients of copies of correspondence include the patient's general medical practitioner, general dental practitioner, social worker, care home manager and any other legitimately interested parties. In each case, a decision needs to be made by the author of any correspondence as to the appropriateness of copying in such individuals. Consent to do this must be sought from the patient.

The National Health Service Plan has made a commitment that patients should be able to receive copies of clinicians' letters about themselves as of right. Consideration should be given to this principle, and also to the provision of any copies in an accessible format according to that patient's needs.

**Hospital NHS Trust (Dental Hospital)**

Tel No: 0123 456789     **Letter of referral**     Fax No: 0123 567890

| | | |
|---|---|---|
| ☐ Conservation | ☐ Child Dental | **X** Oral Surgery |
| ☐ Orthodontics | ☐ Radiology | ☐ Sedation |
| ☐ Periodontics | ☐ Oral Medicine | ☐ Prosthodontics |

---

Title:   *Mr*                             Sex:   M ~~/F~~

Surname:   *Smith*            First Name:   *John*

Surname at Birth:   *N/A*      Middle name: *Albert*

Address:   *1 The Street, City*       Date of Birth: *6 June 46*

Postcode:   *AB1 2CD*        NHS Number: *123-456-7890*

Telephone    Home: *0123 567 8910*     Mobile:     *0789 101112*

               Work: *01223 456 7890*

Ambulance Patient:   ~~Y~~/ N

---

| **Registered GDP** | **Registered GMP** |
|---|---|
| Name: *Dr A N Other* | Name: *Dr G Practice* |
| Address: *The Dental Practice, City* | Address: *The Surgery, City* |
| Postcode: *AB2 3EF* | Postcode: *AB3 4GH* |
| Telephone No: *45 6789* | Telephone No: *456 7890* |

---

Dear Professor Smith, TWO WEEK RULE REFERRAL

I am writing to refer the above named patient for assessment and subsequent treatment. Mr Smith presented today, as a new patient, complaining of pain to LEFT face over a period of several weeks, giving a vague history. On examination Mr Smith was noted to have a swollen lymph node in his neck. Mouth opening was limited to about 2 fingers. Intra-orally there was a large hard ulcer with an erythematous margin in his LEFT retromolar region, approximately 3 cm in diameter. The adjacent teeth, 37 and 36, were both mobile, a radiograph taken at this visit showing a 2 x 1 cm radiolucency with a poorly defined margin in the lower left molar region (enclosed).

The patient had a heart attack in 2009 and has stable angina. In addition he has COPD. Current medication includes aspirin, atenolol, diltiazem, salbutamol and a GTN (used rarely). Mr Smith is retired, lives with his daughter, smokes 30 cigarettes per day and drinks 40 units of alcohol per week.

Mr Smith will require ambulance transport, although he is able to walk short distances unaided.

I would be grateful if you would see this patient as a matter of urgency, as I suspect that this may be an oral cancer.

Please confirm receipt of this fax referral, I will send the original in the post today.

Signed:     *A N Other*        Print Name:   A.N. Other     Date:   1 January 11

Please return to: Records Department, Dental Hospital, Hospital NHS Trust, City, AB1 2CD

**Figure 10.2** An example of a referral letter for a patient being referred under the 2-week rule. It is important that it is clearly labelled as such.

It is felt that by copying letters between professionals to patients there are several potential benefits. These include: increasing the trust between the two parties; producing better informed patients who can then be better able to make decisions about themselves; improve compliance by increasing the patients understanding of a condition; making patients better prepared for a consultation appointment and may even serve to reinforce health promotion messages regarding self-care and lifestyles.

Where a patient is not legally responsible for their own care (for instance, a young child or 'looked after child'), then letters should be copied to the person with legal responsibility (e.g. a parent or legal guardian).

Letters should *not* be copied to patients in the situations summarised in Box 10.3.

---

**Box 10.3   Situations in which letters should not normally be copied to patients**

- The patient has indicated that they do not wish to receive a copy.
- The clinician feels it may cause harm to the patient.
- The letter contains information about a third party who has not given consent.
- There are specific safeguards for confidentiality in place, e.g. if a letter contains particularly sensitive information such as HIV status.

---

Once the decision has been made with regard to whom to copy a letter, this should be documented by the letters 'CC' at the bottom of the letter followed by the list of those it has been copied to. This informs all parties of the recipients of the letter and increases various lines of communication.

## Summary

The following list summarises important principles that should be considered when referring patients:

- Decide whether the referral is necessary and appropriate.
- Try to be specific with regard to whom to refer.
- Refer separate problems via individual referrals.
- Refer promptly.
- Include necessary information. As a minimum:
  - Patient's name, date of birth, address and telephone number
  - Practitioners name, address and telephone number
  - A description of the complaint
- Provide results of further investigations where available.
- Inform the patient that they are being referred and why.

- Indicate the urgency of a referral appropriately.
- Follow specific guidelines for suspected cancers.
- Follow-up the referral.

## Further reading

Standards for dental professionals (2005) General Dental Council, London. Reprinted October 2009. http://www.gdc-uk.org/Dentalprofessionals/ Standards/Pages/default.aspx

Referral guidelines for suspected cancer (2000) Department of Health, London. http://www.dh.gov.uk/en/Publicationsandstatistics/Publications/Publications PolicyAndGuidance/DH_4008746

Referral guidelines for suspected cancer (2005) National Institute of Health and Clinical Excellence, London. Clinical Guideline CG27. http://guidance.nice .org.uk/CG27

# Chapter 11

# Medical Emergencies in the Dental Emergency Clinic – Principles of Management

## M. Greenwood

## Introduction

The commonest medical emergencies seen in the dental emergency clinic are faints. Hypoglycaemia, asthma, anaphylaxis, angina and seizures may also be seen but are less common. All members of the dental team need to be aware of what their role would be in the event of a medical emergency and should be trained appropriately with regular practise sessions.

A thorough history is always important. If a medical condition is identified and medication is normally taken, a check should always be made to ensure that the medication has been taken as usual and its usual level of efficacy.

## Contents of the emergency drug box

Medical emergencies may require equipment, drugs or both in order to manage them effectively and all must be available to use if necessary. Emergency telephone numbers should be known by all members of the team.

Drugs to be included in the emergency drug box are summarised in Table 11.1. The list is based on that given in a Resuscitation Council (UK) document on Medical Emergencies and Resuscitation in Dentistry, the reference to which is given at the end of the chapter.

The Resuscitation Council (UK) recommends that such kits should be standardised throughout the United Kingdom. Drugs ideally should be carried in a pre-filled syringe or kit (Figure 11.1). All drugs should be stored together and ideally in a purpose-designed container.

The optimum route for delivery of emergency drugs is usually the intravenous route but dentists are often inexperienced with this route of delivery.

*Dental Emergencies*, First Edition. Edited by Mark Greenwood and Ian Corbett.
© 2012 Blackwell Publishing Ltd. Published 2012 by Blackwell Publishing Ltd.

**Table 11.1** Contents of the emergency drug box and routes of administration.

| Drug | Route of administration |
|---|---|
| Oxygen | Inhalation |
| Glyceryl trinitrate spray (400 μg per actuation) | Sublingual |
| Dispersible aspirin (300 mg) | Oral (chewed) |
| Adrenaline injection (1:1000, 1 mg/mL) | Intramuscular |
| Salbutamol aerosol inhaler (100 μg per actuation) | Inhalation |
| Glucagon injection (1 mg) | Intramuscular/subcutaneous |
| Oral glucose solution/gel (GlucoGel®)[a] | Oral |
| Midazolam 10 mg or 5 mg/mL (buccal or intra-nasal) | Infiltration/inhalation |

[a]Alternatives:
Two teaspoons of sugar/three sugar lumps
200 mL milk
Non-diet Coca-cola® 90 mL
Non-diet Lucozade® 50 mL
If necessary, this can be repeated at 10-15 minutes.

As a result of this, formulations have now been developed that allow for other routes to be used, which are much quicker and user-friendly. The intravenous route for emergency drugs is no longer recommended for dental practitioners. Oxygen should always be available, deliverable at adequate flow rates (up to 15 L/min) via a non-rebreathe mask (Figure 11.2). The non-rebreathe mask has a one-way valve that means that oxygen delivery is maximised and inhalation of expired carbon dioxide is minimised.

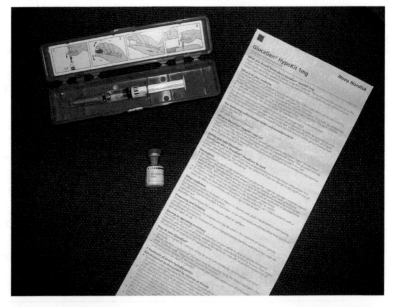

**Figure 11.1** A 'Glucagon Kit' with water for dilution drawn up and powder for reconstitution.

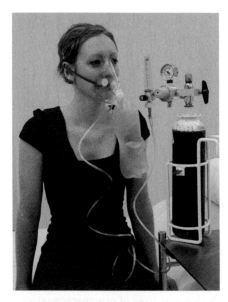

**Figure 11.2** Oxygen being administered via a non-rebreathe mask. Note the reservoir bag and the D type oxygen cylinder.

### Equipment for use in medical emergencies

The Resuscitation Council (UK) have recommended as a minimum the equipment shown in Box 11.1. Named individuals should be nominated to check equipment and this should be carried out at least weekly and the process should be audited.

> ### Box 11.1   Minimum equipment for medical emergency management
>
> - Portable oxygen cylinder (D size) with a flow meter and pressure reduction valve attached to a non-rebreathe mask (Figure 11.2)
> - Oxygen face mask with tubing
> - Oropharyngeal airways – sizes 1, 2, 3 and 4 (Figure 11.3)
> - Pocket mask with port for oxygen
> - Bag and mask apparatus (1 L bag capacity) with oxygen reservoir
> - Well-fitting face masks
> - Portable suction
> - Single-use sterile syringes and needles
> - 'Spacer' device for inhaled bronchodilators
> - Blood glucose measurement device
> - Automated external defibrillator (AED) – see Figure 11.5
>
> *Source:* Adapted from Resuscitation Council (UK).

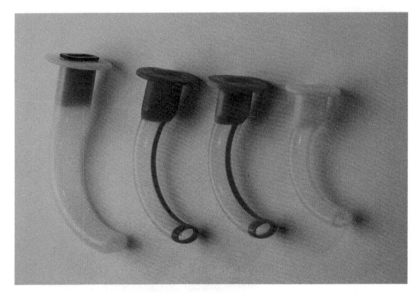

**Figure 11.3** Various sizes of oro-pharyngeal airway.

It is a public expectation that AEDs (see later) should be available in the healthcare environment and dentistry is not considered an exception. All emergency medical equipment should be latex free and single use wherever possible.

## The 'ABCDE' approach to an emergency patient

Medical emergencies can often be prevented by early recognition. An abnormal patient colour, pulse rate or breathing can signal some impending emergencies.

It is important to have a systematic approach to an acutely ill patient and to remain calm. The principles are summarised in the 'ABCDE' approach (Box 11.2).

---

**Box 11.2    The ABCDE approach to an emergency patient**

A: Airway
B: Breathing
C: Circulation
D: Disability (or neurological status)
E: Exposure (in dental practice, to facilitate placement of AED paddles) or appropriately exposing parts to be examined, for example to observe a rash

---

Ensure that the environment is safe. It is important to call for help at a very early stage. Continuous reappraisal of the patient's condition should be carried out and the airway must always be the starting point for this. Without appropriate oxygen delivery, all other management steps will be ultimately futile. It is important to assess the success or otherwise of manoeuvres or treatments given, bearing in mind that treatments may take time to work.

Talking to the patient may give important information about the problem (for example, the patient who cannot speak or tells you that they have chest pain). If the patient is unresponsive, the patient should be shaken and asked 'Are you all right?'. If they do not respond at all, have no pulse and show 'no signs of life' they may have had a cardiac arrest and should be managed as described later. 'Signs of life' refers to breathing and circulation (see later). If they respond in a breathless manner, they should be asked 'Are you choking?'.

## Airway (A)

Airway obstruction is a medical emergency and must be managed quickly and effectively. Usually, a simple method of clearing the airway is all that is needed. A head tilt, chin lift or jaw thrust will open the airway. Patients who are unable to speak are to be feared and establishing a patent airway is vital. It is important to remove any visible foreign bodies, blood or debris and the use of suction may be beneficial. Clearing the mouth should be done with great care using a 'finger sweep' in adults to avoid pushing material further into the upper airway. Simple airway adjuncts, such as an oropharyngeal airway (Figure 11.3) may be used. An impaired airway may be recognised by some of the signs and symptoms summarised in Box 11.3.

> **Box 11.3 Signs of airway obstruction**
>
> - Inability to speak or complete sentences
> - 'Paradoxical' movement of chest and abdomen ('see-saw' respiration)
> - Use of accessory muscles of respiration
> - Blue lips and tongue (central cyanosis)
> - No breathing sounds (complete airway obstruction)
> - Gurgling (suggests liquid or semi-solid material in the upper airway)
> - Stridor (inspiratory) - obstruction of larynx or above
> - Wheeze (expiratory) - obstruction of lower airways, e.g. asthma or chronic obstructive pulmonary disease
> - Snoring (the pharynx is partly occluded by the soft palate or tongue)

It is important to administer oxygen at high concentration (up to 15 L/min) via a well-fitting face mask with a port for oxygen. Even patients with chronic obstructive pulmonary disease who retain carbon dioxide should be given a high concentration of oxygen. Such patients may depend on hypoxic drive to stimulate respiration but in the short-term a high concentration of oxygen will do no harm.

## Breathing (B) and circulation (C)

A clinician should look, listen and feel for signs of respiratory distress:

- *Look* for chest movement with the airway open.
- *Listen* for breath sounds at the victim's mouth.
- *Feel* for air on the rescuer's cheek with the rescuer's head turned against the patient's mouth.
- This should be done for no more than 10 seconds to determine normal breathing.
- If there is any doubt as to whether breathing is normal, action should be as if it is not normal, i.e. commence cardiopulmonary resuscitation (CPR).

A victim may be barely breathing or gasping in the first few minutes after cardiac arrest and this should not be mistaken for normal breathing. Agonal gasps refer to abnormal breathing present in up to 40% of victims of cardiac arrest. Therefore, CPR should be carried out if the victim is unconscious (un-responsive) and not breathing normally. Agonal gasps should not delay the start of CPR as they are not normal breathing.

*If the patient is breathing normally, the patient should*:

- Be turned into the recovery position (essentially on their side – best learnt as a practical exercise).
- Send for help.
- Ensure that breathing continues.

*If the patient is not breathing normally*:

- Ensure that help is summoned (may necessitate leaving the victim) but in a dental setting the practitioner should not be working alone.
- Start chest compressions:
  o Place the heel of one hand in the centre of the victim's chest and the other hand on top of the first hand.
  o Interlock the fingers of both hands – do not apply pressure over the ribs, upper abdomen or the lower end of the sternum.
  o The rescuer should be positioned vertically above the victim's chest. With straight arms the sternum should be depressed 5-6 cm.

- ○ After each compression all the pressure should be released so that the rib cage recoils to its rest position but the hands should be maintained in contact with the sternum.
- ○ The rate should be approximately 100–200 times per minute (a little less than 2 compressions per second).
- After 30 compressions, the airway should be opened using a head tilt and chin lift and two rescue breaths should be given. This may be carried out using a bag and mask or mouth to mouth (with the nostrils closed between thumb and index finger) or mouth to mask.
- Practical skills are best learnt on a resuscitation course but certain principles are given below:
  - ○ Inflations should make the chest rise. About 1 second should be taken to do this.
  - ○ The chest should be allowed to fall whilst maintaining the airway. Two rescue breaths should be given.
  - ○ Hands should be returned to the sternum without delay to continue the chest compressions in a ratio of 30:2.
- Only stop to recheck the patient if normal breathing starts, otherwise resuscitation should be continuous until:
  - ○ qualified help takes over;
  - ○ the rescuer becomes exhausted.

*If rescue breaths do not make the chest rise:*

- Check for a visible obstruction in the mouth and remove, if possible.
- Make sure that the head tilt and chin lift are adequate.
- Do not waste time attempting more than two breaths each time before continuing chest compressions.

Carrying out these manoeuvres is tiring and if there is more than one rescuer CPR should be alternated between them every 2 minutes. The algorithm for adult basic life support is given in Figure 11.4.

### Factors to consider in assessing circulation (C)

Circulatory assessment should never delay the start of CPR. Simple observations to make a gross assessment of circulatory efficiency are given in Box 11.4. By far the most common cause of a collapse that is circulatory in origin is the simple faint (vaso-vagal syncope). A rapid recovery can be expected in these cases if the patient is laid flat and the legs raised. Prompt management is required, however, as cerebral hypoxia has devastating consequences if prolonged. Other causes than a faint must be considered if recovery does not happen rapidly.

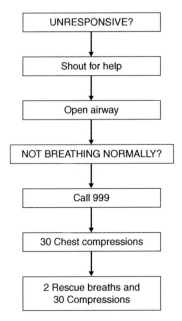

**Figure 11.4** Algorithm for basic life support (adult). Reproduced with permission from Resuscitation Council (UK).

---

**Box 11.4   Simple methods of assessing the circulation**

*Signs*

- Are the patient's hands blue or pink, cool or warm?
- What is the capillary refill time?[a]
- Pulse rate (carotid or radial artery), rhythm and strength

*Symptoms*

- Is there a history of chest pain/does the patient report chest pain?

---

[a]If pressure is applied to the fingernail to produce blanching, the colour should return in less than 2 seconds in a normal patient. Remember that local causes such as a cold environment could also delay the response.

Checking the carotid pulse should only be carried out by practitioners proficient in doing this. The latest guidelines highlight the need to identify agonal gasps (as well as the absence of breathing) as a sign to commence CPR and lay no particular emphasis on checking the carotid pulse.

Once A, B and C are secured, persisting problems should be considered by an appraisal of 'D and E', as discussed in the succeeding sections.

## Disability (D)

Disability refers to an assessment of the neurological status of the patient. In this context, primarily, it refers to the level of consciousness (in trauma patients, a more widespread neurological examination by competent personnel is required). Hypoxia or hypercapnia (increased blood levels of carbon dioxide) are possible causes, together with certain sedative or analgesic drugs.

It is important to exclude hypoxia or hypotension. Attention to the airway, giving supplemental oxygen and supporting the patient's circulation (by lying them supine and raising their legs) will in many cases solve the problem. All unconscious patients who are breathing and have a pulse should be placed in the recovery position if they are unable to maintain their own airway.

A rapid gross assessment can be made of a patient's level of consciousness using the AVPU method: are they Alert?, do they respond to Vocal stimuli? do they respond to Painful stimuli? or are they Unresponsive?

A lapse into unconsciousness may be due to hypoglycaemia – if the blood glucose level is less than 3 mmol/L as checked by a glucose measuring device.

## Exposure (E)

Exposure refers to loosening or removal of some of the patient's clothes. For example, for the application of defibrillator paddles in dental practice or if the patient has been involved in a traumatic incident (usually, in hospital), for examination purposes. It is important to bear in mind the patient's dignity as well as the potential for clinically significant heat loss.

## Cardiac arrest – other considerations

Cardiac arrest can occur for a variety of reasons, which are summarised in Box 11.5.

It has been suggested that cardiopulmonary resuscitation can be performed effectively in the dental chair, but it is important to check that this is the case in any clinical setting.

---

### Box 11.5  Possible causes of cardiac arrest

- Arrhythmia (most common type ventricular fibrillation or VF)
- Myocardial infarction (may lead to an arrhythmia)
- Choking
- Bleeding
- Drug overdose
- Hypoxia

## Use of defibrillation

Defibrillation is the term that refers to the termination of fibrillation. It is achieved by administering a controlled electrical shock to the heart that may restore an organised rhythm enabling the heart to contract effectively. It is now well recognised that early defibrillation is important. Ventricular fibrillation (VF) is the most common cause of cardiac arrest in an adult. The heart is unable to contract effectively and unable to sustain its function as a pump. The only effective treatment for VF is defibrillation and the sooner the shock is given, the greater the chance of survival.

The provision of defibrillation has been made easier by the development of AEDs (Figure 11.5). AEDs are sophisticated, reliable, safe, computerised devices that use voice and visual prompts to guide rescuers and are suitable for use by lay people and healthcare professionals. The device analyses the victim's heart rhythm, determines the need for a shock and then delivers a shock. The AED algorithm is given in Figure 11.6. CPR should not be interrupted/delayed to set up the AED.

### Placement of AED pads

Use of the AED is a skill that needs practical training and experience. The victim's chest must be sufficiently exposed. Excessive chest hair can stop the pads adhering properly and if markedly so must be rapidly removed, if possible. Razors are available in some AED kits. Resuscitation should never be delayed for this reason, however.

One pad should be placed to the right of the sternum below the clavicle and the other in the left side mid-axillary line, centred on the fifth intercostal space. This electrode works best if orientated vertically. This position should be clear of breast tissue. Although most AED pads are labelled or carry a picture of their position, it does not matter if they are reversed.

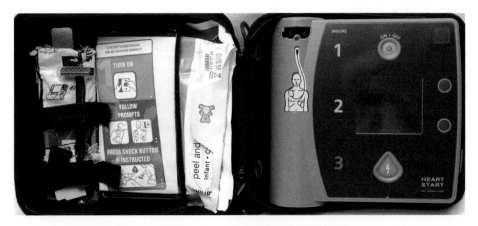

**Figure 11.5** An automated external defibrillator machine.

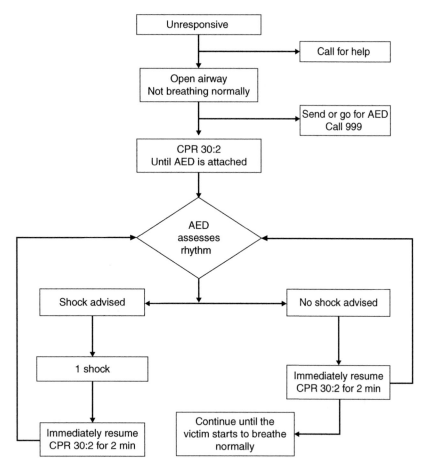

**Figure 11.6** The adult automated external defibrillator algorithm. Reproduced with permission from Resuscitation Council (UK), 2010.

## Principles of management after the initial treatment of a medical emergency

If the practitioner feels competent and confident that the emergency has been managed satisfactorily and the patient is stable, they should still not be allowed to leave the hospital unaccompanied or be allowed to drive a motor vehicle. The decision will be easier to take in some circumstances than others. For example, in cases of the simple faint patients will usually be discharged home and indeed it may be possible to complete planned treatment. The patient who has an angina attack in the surgery, responds very quickly to their normal glyceryl trinitrate and who has a clear history of similar episodes and makes a complete recovery will similarly usually be well enough to be allowed home.

If a patient remains unwell or there is any doubt at all, they should undergo assessment by a medical practitioner. Before any transfer is made, the patient's condition should be stabilised so long as that does not delay ongoing treatment. It is important that a verbal and written summary is given to the receiving team so that treatment that has been undertaken is made clear. A good example is documenting the fact that a patient has been given aspirin or undergone dental surgery making them prone to haemorrhage that may influence the decision to give anti-thrombolytic therapy.

## Conclusions

It is important that dental practitioners have a sound awareness of the principles of management of medical emergencies. More detailed management scenarios are given in Chapter 12. Ultimately, however, the management of all situations depends on adherence to the basic principles outlined in this chapter as ultimately other strategies will prove futile unless this is done.

## Further reading

Medical Emergencies and Resuscitation Standards for Clinical Practice and Training for Dental Practitioners and Dental Care Professionals in General Dental Practice - A Statement from the Resuscitation Council (UK) July 2006. Revised June 2011.
Resuscitation Guidelines 2010.
Resuscitation Council (UK), October 2010.

# Chapter 12

# Examples of Specific Medical Emergency Situations

## M. Greenwood

## Introduction

The general principles of management of medical emergencies were discussed in Chapter 11. This chapter concentrates on specific medical emergencies. The practitioner dealing with specific emergencies must not lose sight of the need to act in accordance with basic principles and be prepared to revisit them if the patient response to treatment is not satisfactory.

Specific emergencies that may arise in dental practice are listed in Box 12.1. Their signs, symptoms and management will be discussed.

---

**Box 12.1  A summary of medical emergencies that may be encountered in a dental emergency clinic**

- Vasovagal syncope (faint)
- Hyperventilation/'panic attack'
- Acute asthma attack
- Angina/myocardial infarction
- Epileptic seizures
- Diabetic emergencies
- Allergies/hypersensitivity reactions
- Choking and aspiration
- Adrenal insufficiency
- Cardiac arrest (see Chapter 11)

---

*Dental Emergencies*, First Edition. Edited by Mark Greenwood and Ian Corbett.
© 2012 Blackwell Publishing Ltd. Published 2012 by Blackwell Publishing Ltd.

## Vasovagal syncope (simple faint)

The 'simple faint' is the most common medical emergency to be seen in dental practice and results in loss of consciousness due to inadequate cerebral perfusion. It is a reflex that is mediated by autonomic nerves leading to widespread vasodilatation in the splanchnic and skeletal vessels and bradycardia resulting in diminished cerebral perfusion. Fainting can be precipitated by pain or emotional stress, changes in posture or hypoxia. Some patients are more prone to fainting than others and it is wise to treat fainting-prone patients in the supine position.

A similar clinical picture may be seen in 'carotid sinus syndrome'. Mild pressure on the neck in such patients (usually, the elderly) leads to a vagal reaction producing syncope. This situation may progress to bradycardia or even cardiac arrest.

### Fainting – signs and symptoms

- Patient feels faint/light headed/dizzy
- Pallor, sweating
- Pulse rate slows
- Low blood pressure
- Nausea and/or vomiting
- Loss of consciousness

### Fainting – treatment

- Lay the patient flat and raise the legs – recovery will normally be rapid.
- A patent airway must be maintained.
- If recovery is delayed, oxygen should be administered and other causes of loss of consciousness be considered.

## Hyperventilation

Hyperventilation is a more common emergency than is often thought. When hyperventilation persists, it can become extremely distressing to the patient. Anxiety is the principal precipitating factor.

### Hyperventilation – signs and symptoms

- Anxiety
- Light headedness
- Dizziness
- Weakness
- Paraesthesia
- Tetany (see below)

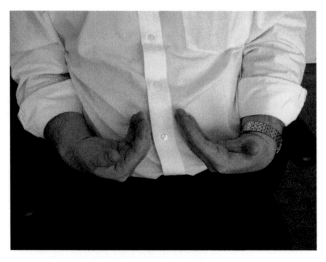

**Figure 12.1** A demonstration of carpal spasm.

- Chest pain and/or palpitations
- Breathlessness

### Hyperventilation – treatment

A calm and sympathetic approach from the practitioner is important. The diagnosis, particularly in the early stages, is not always as obvious as it may seem:

- Exclude other causes for the symptoms.
- Encourage the patient to rebreathe their own exhaled air to increase the amount of inhaled carbon dioxide – a paper bag placed over nose and mouth allows this.
- If no paper bag is handy, the patient's cupped hands would be a (less satisfactory) alternative.

Hyperventilation leads to carbon dioxide being 'washed out' of the body producing an alkalosis. If hyperventilation persists, carpal (hand) and pedal (foot) spasm (tetany) may be seen (Figure 12.1). Re-breathing exhaled air increases inspired carbon dioxide levels and helps to return the situation to normal.

## Asthma

Asthma is a potentially life-threatening condition and should always be taken seriously. An attack may be precipitated by exertion, anxiety, infection or exposure to an allergen. It is important in the history to get some idea of the severity of attacks. Clues include the precipitating factors, effectiveness of medication, hospital admissions due to asthma and the use of systemic steroids.

It is important that asthmatic patients bring their usual inhaler(s) with them – if the inhaler has not been brought it must be in the emergency kit or treatment should be deferred. If the asthma is in a particularly severe phase, elective treatment may be best postponed. Drugs that may be prescribed by dental practitioners, particularly non-steroidal anti-inflammatory drugs, may worsen asthma and, therefore, are best avoided.

## Asthma – signs and symptoms

- Breathlessness (rapid respiration – more than 25 breaths per minute)
- Expiratory wheezing
- Use of accessory muscles of respiration
- Tachycardia

## Signs and symptoms of life-threatening asthma

- Cyanosis or slow respiratory rate (less than 8 breaths per minute)
- Bradycardia
- Decreased level of consciousness/confusion

## Asthma – treatment

- Most attacks will respond to the patient's own inhaler, usually salbutamol (may need to repeat after 2–3 minutes).
- If no rapid response, or features of severe asthma, call an ambulance.
- A medical assessment should be arranged for patients who require additional doses of bronchodilator to end an attack.
- A spacer device may need to be used if patient has difficulty using the inhaler.
- If the patient is distressed or shows any of the signs of life-threatening asthma, urgent transport to hospital should be arranged.
- High-flow oxygen should be given whilst awaiting transfer. Four to six actuations from the salbutamol inhaler via a spacer device should be used and repeated every 10 minutes. In the British National Formulary, a technique is described for a 'home made' spacer device. A hole can be cut out the base of a paper or plastic cup. The mouthpiece of the inhaler is pushed through this. The open end of the cup can then be applied to the mouth when the inhaler is activated.
- If asthma is part of a more generalised anaphylactic reaction, or *in extremis*, an intramuscular injection of adrenaline should be given (see Section 'Anaphylaxis').

All patients, including those who have chronic obstructive pulmonary disease, should be given high-flow oxygen as even if these patients are dependent on 'hypoxic drive' to stimulate their respiration, they will come to no harm in the short-term.

## Cardiac chest pain

Most patients who suffer chest pain from a cardiac cause in the dental surgery are likely to have a previous history of cardiac disease. The history is clearly important and if a patient uses medication to control known angina they should have brought this with them or it should be readily to hand in the emergency kit. Similarly, it is important that the patient has taken their normal medication on the day of their appointment.

Classically, the pain of angina is described as a crushing or band-like tightness of the chest, which may radiate to the left arm or mandible. There are many variations, however. The pain of myocardial infarction (MI) will often be similar to that of angina but more severe and, unlike angina, will not be relieved by GTN. In cases of angina, the patient should use their glyceryl trinitrate (GTN) spray, which will usually remove the symptoms. Dental treatment may be best left until another day if there is an attack, according to the practitioner's discretion. More severe chest pain always warrants postponement of treatment and an ambulance should be called.

Features that make chest pain unlikely to be cardiac in origin are: pains that last less than 30 seconds, however severe; stabbing pains; well-localised left submammary pain and pains that continually vary in location. Chest pain that improves on stopping exertion is more likely to be cardiac in origin than one that is not related. Pleuritic pain is sharp in character, well localised and worse on inspiration.

Oesophagitis can produce a retrosternal pain that worsens on bending or lying down. A complicating factor in differentiation from cardiac chest pain is that GTN, due to action on the muscle of the oesophagus, may ease the pain.

Musculoskeletal pain is generally accompanied by tenderness to palpation in the affected region. As mentioned earlier, hyperventilation may produce chest pain. A list of possible causes of chest pain is given in Box 12.2.

---

### Box 12.2 Chest pain – possible causes

- Angina
- Myocardial infarction
- Pleuritic, e.g. pulmonary embolism
- Musculoskeletal
- Oesophageal reflux
- Hyperventilation
- Gall bladder and pancreatic disease

It is clearly important to exclude angina and MI in the patient complaining of chest pain. If in doubt, treat as cardiac pain until proven otherwise.

## Myocardial infarction – signs and symptoms

- Severe, crushing chest pain, which may radiate to the shoulders and down the arms (particularly the left arm) and into the mandible.
- Shortness of breath.
- The skin becomes pale and clammy.
- Pulse becomes weak and patient may become hypotensive.
- Often, there will be nausea and vomiting.

Not all patients fit this picture and may exhibit only some of the signs and symptoms mentioned in the preceeding text.

## Myocardial infarction – treatment

- The practitioner should remain calm and be a reassuring presence.
- Call emergency number.
- Most patients will be best managed in the sitting position.
- Patients who feel faint should be laid flat.
- Give high-flow oxygen (15 L/min).
- Give sublingual GTN spray.
- Give 300 mg aspirin orally to be chewed (if no allergy) - ensure that when handing over to the receiving ambulance crew that they are made aware of this as thrombolytic therapy is given by some ambulance crews.
- A patient who has had surgical dental treatment should be highlighted to the ambulance crew as any significant risk of haemorrhage may affect the decision to use thrombolytic therapy
- If the patient becomes unresponsive, the practitioner should check for 'signs of life' (breathing and circulation) and start cardiac pulmonary ressusication.

## Epileptic seizures

The history will usually reveal the fact that a patient has epilepsy. A history should obtain information with regard to the nature of any seizures, their frequency and degree of control. The type and efficacy of medication should be determined. Signs and symptoms vary considerably.

## Epilepsy – signs and symptoms

- The patient may have an 'aura' or premonition that a seizure is about to occur.
- Tonic phase - loss of consciousness, patient becomes rigid and falls and becomes cyanosed.
- Clonic phase - jerking movements of the limbs, tongue may be bitten.

- Urinary incontinence, frothing at the mouth.
- The seizure often gradually abates after a few minutes but the patient may remain unconscious and may remain confused after consciousness has been regained
- Hypoglycaemia may present as a fit and should be considered (including in epileptic patients). Therefore, blood glucose measurement at an early stage is wise.

In patients with a marked bradycardia (less than 40 beats per minute), the blood pressure may drop to such an extent that it causes transient cerebral hypoxia leading to a brief fit. This is not a true fit and represents a vasovagal episode.

## Epilepsy – treatment of a fit

The decision to give medication should be made if seizures are prolonged (with active convulsions for 5 minutes or more (status epilepticus) or seizures occurring in quick succession). If possible, high-flow oxygen should be administered. The possibility of the patient's airway becoming occluded should be constantly remembered, and therefore, the airway must be protected:

- As far as possible, ensure safety of the patient and practitioner (do not attempt to restrain).
- Midazolam given via the buccal or intra-nasal route (10 mg for adults). The buccal preparation is marketed as 'Epistatus' (10 mg/mL) (Figure 12.2).

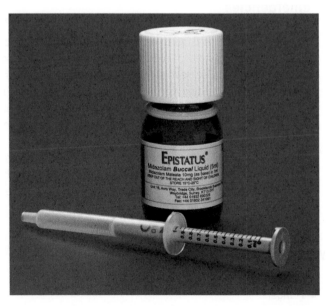

**Figure 12.2** Buccal/intra-nasal midazolam. The solution in the bottle is drawn up in the syringe provided, which is calibrated into 0.1 mL increments.

- For children:
  - o Child 1-5 years-5 mg
  - o Child 5-10 years-7.5 mg
  - o Child more than 10 years-10 mg
- The parents of some children with poorly controlled epilepsy will carry rectal diazepam. As part of pre-treatment preparation, it is wise to arrange with the parent for them to be on hand to administer this should a fit arise.
- In the absence of rapid response to treatment, call an ambulance.

Criteria for sending a patient with epilepsy to hospital who has had a seizure have been developed by the National Institute for Health and Clinical Excellence and are summarised in Box 12.3.

---

**Box 12.3   NICE guidelines relating to onward referral after a fit**

- Status epilepticus
- High risk of recurrence of fits
- First fit
- Difficulty in monitoring the patient's condition

---

## Diabetic emergencies

The history should be used to assess the degree of diabetic control achieved by the patient. A history of recurrent hypoglycaemic episodes and markedly varying blood glucose levels (from the patient's measurements) suggest that a patient attending for dental treatment is more likely to develop hypoglycaemia. It is wise to treat diabetic patients first on any list and ensure that they have had their normal medication and something to eat prior to attending.

A dentist in general practice is much more likely to encounter hypoglycaemia than hyperglycaemia, since the latter has a much slower onset. It should be remembered that diabetic control may be adversely affected by oral sepsis, leading to an increased risk of complications.

### Hypoglycaemia – signs and symptoms

- Trembling
- Hunger
- Headache

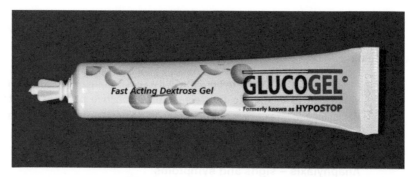

**Figure 12.3** Gluco Gel® for use in a conscious hypoglycaemic patient. The top of the tube can be twisted off and the patient should ingest the entire contents of the tube.

- Sweating
- Slurring of speech
- 'Pins and needles' in lips and tongue
- Aggression and/or confusion
- Seizures
- Unconsciousness

**Hypoglycaemia – treatment**

- Lie the patient flat (remember A, B, C).
- If the patient is conscious, give oral glucose (three lumps of sugar or 2-4 teaspoons of sugar) or Gluco Gel® (Figure 12.3).
- If the patient is unconscious, give 1 mg glucagon intramuscularly (or subcutaneously).
- Get medical help.

Patients who do not respond to glucagon (a rarity) or those who have exhausted their supplies of liver glycogen will require 20 mL of intravenous glucose solution (20-50%) and should be managed under medical supervision or by the attending ambulance team. It can take glucagon 5-10 minutes to be effective and the patient's airway must be protected at all times.

Once the patient regains consciousness and has an intact gag reflex, they should be given glucose orally and a high carbohydrate food. If full recovery is achieved and the patient is accompanied, they may be allowed home but should not be allowed to drive. The general medical practitioner should be informed of the event.

The principle of treatment of hyperglycaemia is through intravenous rehydration. This should be carried out under medical supervision and is beyond the scope of this discussion.

## Allergies/hypersensitivity reactions

### Anaphylaxis

Anaphylaxis is a Type I hypersensitivity reaction involving IgE to which free antigen binds leading to the release of vasoactive peptides and histamine. Penicillin and latex are the most likely causes in dentistry. Local anaesthetics are rarely responsible.

#### Anaphylaxis – signs and symptoms
- Itchy rash/erythema.
- Facial flushing or pallor.
- Upper airway (laryngeal) oedema and bronchospasm leading to stridor, wheezing and possibly hoarseness.
- A respiratory arrest may occur leading to cardiac arrest.
- Vasodilatation leading to low blood pressure and collapse, which may progress to cardiac arrest.

#### Anaphylaxis – initial treatment
- The ABCDE approach should be employed while the diagnosis is being made.
- Manage airway and breathing by administering high-flow oxygen.
- Restore blood pressure by lying the patient flat and raising the legs.

In life-threatening anaphylaxis (hoarseness, stridor, cyanosis, dyspnoea, drowsiness, confusion or coma), adrenaline should be administered:

- Administer 0.5 mL of 1 in 1000 adrenaline IM and repeat and 5-minute intervals if no improvement.
- The optimum site for injection is the anterolateral mid-third of the thigh.

Chlorphenamine (antihistamine) and hydrocortisone (steroid) need not be given by non-medical 'first responders'. As a result, the only drug required to

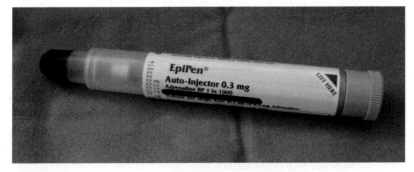

**Figure 12.4** An 'EpiPen' containing 300 µg of adrenaline.

be administered by dental practitioners is adrenaline. The other drugs will be administered by ambulance personnel, if necessary.

Many patients with a history of anaphylactic reactions will carry an 'EpiPen', which contains 300 µg of adrenaline. This may be used if such a patient has an anaphylactic reaction in the dental surgery (Figure 12.4). Variation in the doses of adrenaline that may be given to different age groups are summarised in Box 12.4.

---

**Box 12.4   Intramuscular adrenaline – dose variation with age**

- Adult (or child >12 years) - 500 µg (0.5 mL)
- Child (6-12 years) - 300 µg (0.3 mL)
- Child (<6 years) - 150 µg (0.15 mL)

All refer to IM doses of adrenaline (1:1000).

---

## Angioedema

Angioedema is triggered when mast cells release histamine and other chemicals into the blood producing rapid swelling that may be life-threatening if the airway is involved. It may be precipitated by substances such as latex and penicillin. There is an hereditary component. Signs and symptoms are summarised in Box 12.5.

Hereditary angioedema (HANE) is caused by complement activation resulting from a deficiency of the inhibitor of the enzyme C1 esterase. It is usually inherited as autosomal dominant and may not present until adulthood. C1 esterase inhibitor concentrates are available to supplement the deficiency and should be administered in a hospital setting. Such supplements should be administered prior to dental treatment if such treatment has previously triggered the onset of angioedema.

---

**Box 12.5   Angioedema – signs and symptoms**

- Swelling around eyes, lips, throat and extremities
- Laryngeal oedema and bronchospasm

Acute allergic oedema may develop alone or be associated with anaphylactic reactions.

---

## Choking and aspiration

Prevention is important by the use of rubber dam, instrument chains, mouth sponges, etc. Careful suction of the oral cavity and close observation minimise risk. If a patient is suspected of having aspirated a foreign body, they should be encouraged to cough vigorously in attempt to clear the airway and 'cough up' the object. A foreign body may lead to either mild or severe airway obstruction. Signs and symptoms that can aid in differentiation of the degree of airway obstruction are shown in Box 12.6. In a conscious victim, it is useful to ask the question 'Are you choking?'. An algorithm for the management of a choking patient has been published by the Resuscitation Council (UK) and is given in Figure 12.5.

---

**Box 12.6   Management of a choking victim – signs and symptoms**

*General signs of choking*

- Attack occurs while eating/misplaced dental instrument/restoration.
- Victim may clutch his neck.

*Signs of mild airway obstruction*

Response to question 'Are you choking?'
- Victim speaks and answers 'YES'.

*Other signs*

- Victim is able to speak, cough and breathe.

*Signs of severe airway obstruction*

Response to question 'Are you choking?'
- Victim unable to speak.
- Victim may respond by nodding.

*Other signs*

- Victim unable to breathe.
- Breathing sounds wheezy.
- Attempts at coughing are silent.
- Victim may be unconscious.

*Source:* Adapted from Resuscitation Guidelines 2010 (Resuscitation Council (UK)).

---

The back blows mentioned in the algorithm are delivered by standing to the side of the victim and slightly behind. The chest should be supported with one hand and the victim leant well forwards so that when the obstruction is

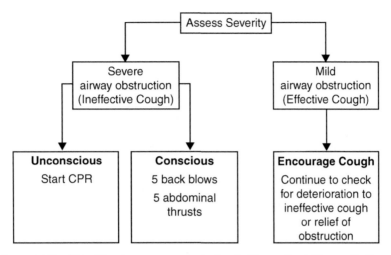

Figure 12.5 Algorithm for management of a choking patient (Resuscitation Council (UK) 2010). Abdominal thrusts should not be used in infants due to the risk of damage to intra-abdominal organs. Reproduced with permission from Resuscitation Council (UK).

dislodged it is expelled from the mouth rather than passing further down the airway. Up to five sharp blows should be given between the shoulder blades with the heel of the other hand. After each back blow, a check should be made to see if the obstruction has been relieved.

If back blows fail, up to five abdominal thrusts should be given (Figure 12.6):

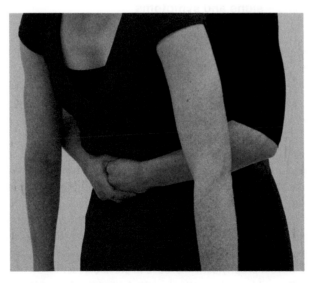

Figure 12.6 Abdominal thrusts. Note that the victim is leaning forwards slightly. The interlocked hands of the rescuer should pull sharply upwards and inwards in an adult patient.

- Stand behind the victim and put both arms around the upper part of their abdomen and lean them forwards.
- The rescuer's fist should be clenched and placed between the umbilicus and lower end of the sternum.
- The clenched fist should be grasped with the other hand and pulled sharply inwards and upwards.
- This should be repeated up to five times.
- The back blows and abdominal thrusts should be continued in a cyclical fashion.

If it is suspected that a foreign body has been inhaled, the patient must be referred for chest radiography. Radiographs will be taken in two planes (postero-anterior and lateral). The foreign body is most likely to be seen in the right lung or right main bronchus as the latter is more vertical than the left. Bronchoscopy or even thoracotomy may be required to retrieve it.

## Adrenal insufficiency

Adrenal crisis may result from adrenocortical hypofunction leading to hypotension, shock and death. It may be precipitated by stress induced by trauma, surgery or infection. It is rare that this would happen as a result of dental treatment and if a patient collapses other causes are much more likely and should be considered first.

### Adrenal crisis – signs and symptoms

- The patient loses consciousness.
- The patient has a rapid, weak or impalpable pulse.
- The blood pressure falls rapidly.

Management involves the use of intravenous hydrocortisone and intravenous fluids. The above is a holding measure only.

It is important in the history to ascertain whether the patient has recently used or is currently using corticosteroids. Some patients carry a 'steroid warning card'. Acute adrenal insufficiency can often be prevented by the administration of a steroid boost prior to treatment. Recent studies have suggested that dental surgery may not require supplementation. More invasive procedures, however, such as oral surgical procedures or the treatment of very apprehensive patients may still require cover. Patients who are systemically unwell (e.g. patients with a significant dental abscess) are also recommended to have a prophylactic increase in steroid dose.

The guidance for patients with Addison's disease is to double the patient's steroid dose before significant dental treatment under local anaesthesia and continue this for 24 hours.

## Adrenal crisis – treatment

- Lie the patient flat and raise their legs.
- Ensure a clear airway and administer oxygen.
- Call an ambulance.

# Stroke

Stroke may be either haemorrhagic or embolic in aetiology but clinically the effects are essentially the same. It is highly unlikely that this situation would arise in the dental emergency clinic but an awareness of basic principles is important. Signs and symptoms vary according to the site of brain damage. There may be loss of consciousness and weakness of limbs on one side of the body. One side of the face may become weak. As stroke causes an upper motor neurone lesion, the forehead muscles of facial expression will be unaffected. Speech may become slurred.

## Stroke – initial management

- The airway should be maintained and an ambulance called.
- High-flow oxygen (15 L/min) should be given.
- The patient should be carefully monitored for any further deterioration.

# Local anaesthetic emergencies

Allergy to local anaesthetic is rare but should be managed as any other case of anaphylaxis. When taken in the context of the number of local anaesthetics administered, complication rates are low. The signs and symptoms in allergy are those of anaphylaxis.

Fainting in association with the injection of local anaesthetic is more common and can usually be avoided by administering the local anaesthetic while the patient is supine.

Intravascular injection of local anaesthetic solution can be avoided by the use of an aspirating syringe. If an intravascular injection does occur, it can induce agitation, drowsiness or confusion with fits and ultimately loss of consciousness. Other potential problems with local analgesia are listed in Box 12.7.

The most common symptoms to be precipitated adversely with local anaesthetic injections are palpitations. These will usually subside with time. It is possible for an interaction to occur with anti-hypertensive drugs to produce hypotension. It is important in these cases to ensure that the airway is maintained, if consciousness becomes impaired. Hypertension may rarely be precipitated and in both cases medical assistance should be obtained. If a cardiovascular event is precipitated, treatment is best deferred. Signs and symptoms, and treatment of an epinephrine overdose is given in Box 12.8.

**Box 12.7   Possible problems with local analgesia**

- Allergy (rare)

*Cardiovascular*

- Palpitations
- Hypotension
- Hypertension
- Myocardial infarction

*Facial palsy or diplopia*
- Provide eye patch.

*Management of a local anaesthetic overdose*
- Stop the procedure.
- Lay the patient flat.
- Administer oxygen.
- If competent, give intravenous fluids and intravenous anticonvulsants.
- Perform basic life support, if needed.

**Box 12.8   Signs, symptoms and treatment of adrenaline overdose**

*Signs of adrenaline overdose*

- Anxiety
- Restlessness
- Headache
- Sweating
- Trembling
- Weakness
- Dizziness
- Pallor
- Respiratory difficulties and palpitations

*Treatment of adrenaline overdose*

- Avoid!
- Stop the procedure.
- Place in a semi-supine or erect position to minimise the increase in cerebral blood pressure.
- Reassurance.
- Administer oxygen if the patient is not hyperventilating.

Temporary facial palsy or diplopia can occur if the local anaesthetic agent is deposited close to the facial nerve or tracks to the orbital contents. The effects wear off as the local anaesthetic effect diminishes and the patient should be reassured. If the temporal and zygomatic branches of the facial nerve are affected, it is important to remember that the patient will be unable to close the ipsilateral eye and the cornea should be protected.

## Needle breakage

Needle breakage is a much less common event since the introduction of single-use needles. It is still a possibility, however, and practitioners should be aware of the action to be taken in such an event. The stages in management are summarised in Box 12.9.

---

**Box 12.9   Steps to be taken in the event of a broken injection needle**

- If the needle tip is visible, remove using artery forceps.

*If the tip of the needle is not visible*

- Inform the patient.
- Arrange immediate referral to maxillofacial surgery.
- Advise the patient against mandibular movement as far as possible.
- Ensure that accurate records are written.
- Inform protection society.

---

Breakages are more likely to occur at the hub of the needle and are more common in those of small diameter. It is only possible to remove the needle using artery forceps if the needle is not inserted to the hilt and as a point of technique, for this reason needles should not be inserted to this degree. If immediate retrieval is not possible, the patient should be informed and referred to a maxillofacial unit. All events should be clearly and accurately documented and the practitioner's medical protection organisation informed.

It is helpful to send the remaining part of the needle with the patient as this will help to illustrate what length is likely to be remaining. Imaging will be carried out at the hospital, first by plain radiography (two views at right angles) and then by computerised tomographic scanning.

If the needle is not retrieved, there is the potential for trismus, pain and dysphagia to develop or the needle could migrate. All of these things depend on where the needle is situated. It can be very difficult, even with the best imaging to locate the fractured needle and therefore in some cases, because the needle is sterile, if there is no reason to suspect that it will migrate, the needle could be left in situ unless complications develop.

## Sedation emergencies

It is very unlikely that intravenous sedation would be administered in the dental emergency clinic. One area in which it may be employed, however, is to facilitate the reduction of a dislocated mandible. Emergencies are relatively rare and are usually avoidable by careful technique. Potential emergencies may relate to overdose, hypoxia or both. Such situations can lead to respiratory arrest if they are not addressed promptly. During any dental treatment under intravenous sedation, the vital signs should be formally monitored.

## Management

The patient should be given no further sedation agent and the airway should be maintained and high-flow oxygen administered. If an overdose of the sedation agent is suspected (usually, a benzodiazepine), the use of the reversal agent flumazenil should be considered, bearing in mind that flumazenil is epileptogenic.

## Problems with haemostasis

Most potential problems with haemostasis will have been highlighted in the medical history and therefore can be anticipated and prevented. Haemorrhage may be classified into three groups, primary, reactionary and secondary. Primary haemorrhage is that which occurs at the time of surgery and reactionary that which occurs a few hours after surgery. A common cause of reactionary haemorrhage is the vasoconstrictor element of adrenaline wearing off leading to haemorrhage. Secondary haemorrhage is that which occurs a few days after the procedure and the commonest cause is infection.

It is important if a bleeding disorder is present that appropriate liaison takes place with a haematologist. A good way of classifying bleeding disorders is into those that are inherited and those that acquired.

Patients with congenital bleeding disorders are best treated in specialist centres as communication between surgeon and haematologist is optimised. Patients with haemophilia A, Christmas disease (factor IX deficiency) or von Willebrand's disease may require replacement therapy before surgery and an anti-fibrinolytic agent (e.g. tranexamic acid) post-operatively. The use of local haemostatic measures such as oxidised cellulose (Surgicel®) should be considered with suturing extraction sockets. Agents such as Surgicel are resorbable. Bone wax is a useful method of arresting blood that is persistently oozing from a bony surface but should be used sparingly as there is a risk of foreign body granuloma development.

Acquired bleeding disorders may result from medication or underlying systemic disease. It is unusual in contemporary practice to stop aspirin treatment before dental surgery. If for any reason aspirin is stopped, this should be done 10 days before surgery as its effect on platelets is irreversible and time is needed to allow some replacement of the platelet population. If aspirin is continued, local haemostatic measures is usually all that is required. Other anti-platelet drugs such as clopidogrel and dipyridamole likewise can be continued and local haemostatic measures applied.

It is now considered that patients who are taking warfarin are at higher risk of an adverse thromboembolic event if this is withdrawn than significant bleeding after dental surgery if it is continued. It has also been suggested that stopping warfarin might lead to a rebound hypercoaguable state thereby increasing the risk of thromboembolism still further.

Patients taking warfarin should have their international normalised ratio (INR) measured before any surgical procedure. This can now be performed in the dental surgery using a finger-prick sample. The normal therapeutic INR for patients taking warfarin is 2–3, except for those with cardiac valve replacements in whom the range is 2.5–3.5.

In the United Kingdom, current advice is that most surgical procedures in dentistry, such as extractions and simple minor oral surgical procedures, may be carried out without alteration of warfarin if the INR is 4 or less (see Appendix 3). If the INR is greater than 4, liaison with the physician who prescribed the warfarin is important as it may need to be temporarily stopped. If this was the case, it is usually stopped 2 days before the procedure and restarted on the evening of the day of procedure. It is not essential to avoid regional block anaesthesia in these patients but preferable if possible. In all patients taking warfarin, local measures of achieving haemostasis should be employed. Patients taking warfarin (or other prospective surgical patients) who have concurrent medical problems as listed in Box 12.10, should not be treated without consultation with the patient's physician.

---

**Box 12.10   Systemic conditions that may lead to problems with haemostasis**

- Liver impairment and/or alcoholism
- Chronic kidney disease
- Thrombocytopaenia, haemophilia or other haemostatic disorder
- Patients undergoing cytotoxic medication or radiotherapy

---

Patients undergoing heparin therapy may be encountered. The most common group is probably patients who are heparinised to facilitate haemodialysis as a result of (usually, chronic) kidney disease. Heparinisation is undertaken usually three times per week but because of the short half-life of heparin (around 5 hours) dental treatment can be carried safely in the days between dialysis. If a heparinised patient required emergency surgical dental treatment, the effects of heparin can be reversed by protamine sulphate but its use should only be done under the supervision of a physician.

Patients may be undergoing treatment with one of the low-molecular-weight heparin agents, for example tinzaparin. Unlike warfarin therapy, which can be monitored using the INR or conventional heparin therapy monitored by the activated partial thromboplastin time, the effects of low-molecular-weight heparin cannot be monitored in this way. Usually, local haemostatic measures are all that is required after dental surgery on this group of patients.

The anti-fibrinolytic agent, tranexamic acid, can reduce post-operative bleeding in anticoagulated patients. Its primary action is to block the binding of plasminogen and plasmin to fibrin, thereby preventing fibrinolysis. It has been suggested that tranexamic acid mouthwash as 4.8% preparation is effective but has to be made up on an individual patient basis.

## Medication and haemostasis

Some drugs that dental practitioners can prescribe will interact with anticoagulants. Analgesics such as aspirin, diclofenac, ibuprofen and long-term use of paracetamol are all examples. Anti-microbials such as those of the penicillin group can increase the prothrombin time in warfarinised patients but this is unusual. Erythromycin enhances the anticoagulant effect of warfarin and nicoumalone by reducing their metabolism. Combined use of these drugs is not absolutely contraindicated but monitoring of such patients is required. The interaction between warfarin and metronidazole is clinically important as it inhibits the metabolism of warfarin. Tetracycline may enhance the effect of warfarin and the other coumarin anticoagulants. Even after topical use, the anti-fungal agent miconazole can enhance the effects of warfarin and lead to catastrophic bleeding. In contrast to the drugs mentioned so far, carbamazepine may reduce the effect of warfarin as its metabolism is increased.

It is important that patients taking warfarin who require a prescription are not prescribed drugs that have a documented interaction. The current British National Formulary or equivalent publication should be consulted.

## Patients with liver problems

Patients with liver failure can be difficult to evaluate in respect of the risk of post-surgical bleeding. A relatively small elevation of the prothrombin time can suggest significant liver damage. The intravenous injection of vitamin K may be required (but only after advice from a haematologist). Fresh frozen plasma will lower the prothrombin time and platelet transfusion may address both qualitative and quantitative problems.

Patients with hepatic problems are potentially at risk when opioid analgesics are prescribed and sedatives such as diazepam. Smaller doses should be used for drugs that are metabolised by the liver. The use of paracetamol should be avoided altogether in the presence of significant hepatic impairment.

## Conclusions

Prompt appropriate management deals with medical emergencies effectively. It is important that each member of the dental team knows what their role should be in the event of a medical emergency. Training should be updated regularly and at least on an annual basis.

## Further reading

Resuscitation Guidelines 2010.
Resuscitation Council (UK), October 2010.
Epilepsy. National Institute for Health and Clinical Excellence. Clinical Guideline CG20. October 2004.

# Appendix 1
# Normal Reference Ranges

Laboratories vary with regard to normal reference ranges but the following are indicative values:

| Basic haematology values | | |
|---|---|---|
| Haemoglobin | Men | 13-18 g/dL |
| | Women | 11.5-16 g/dL |
| Mean cell volume | | 76-96 fL |
| Platelets | | 150-400 × 10$^9$/L |
| White cells | | 4-11 × 10$^9$/L |
| Neutrophils | | 40-75% |
| Lymphocytes | | 20-45% |
| Eosinophils | | 1-6% |
| **Urea and electrolytes** | | |
| Sodium | | 135-145 mmol/L |
| Potassium | | 3.5-5 mmol/L |
| Creatinine | | 70-150 $\mu$mol/L |
| Urea | | 2.5-6.7 mmol/L |
| Calcium | | 2.12-2.65 mmol/L |
| Albumin | | 35-50 g/L |
| Proteins | | 60-80 g/L |
| **Liver function tests** | | |
| Bilirubin | | 3-17 $\mu$mol/L |
| Alanine aminotransferase | | 3-35 units/L |
| Aspartate transaminase | | 3-35 units/L |
| Alkaline phosphatase | | 30-300 units/L |
| **Other** | | |
| C-reactive protein | | <10 mg/L |
| Erythrocyte sedimentation rate | | 0-6 mm in 1 hr normal |
| | | >20 mm in 1 hr abnormal |

*Dental Emergencies*, First Edition. Edited by Mark Greenwood and Ian Corbett.
© 2012 Blackwell Publishing Ltd. Published 2012 by Blackwell Publishing Ltd.

# Appendix 2
# Changes in Vital Signs in Patients with Infection

| | | Changes associated with infection | |
|---|---|---|---|
| | Normal range | Mild to moderate | Serious |
| Oral temperature (°C) | 35.5-37.5 | 37.5-39.5 | Above 40 |
| Pulse (beats/min) | 60-80 | 90-100 | Above 100 |
| Blood pressure (mmHg) | Systolic 120-140 Diastolic 60-90 | No change | May fall (shock) |
| Respiration | | | |
| Airway | Clear | Clear | Obstructed |
| Rate (resps/min) | 12-18 | 18-20 | Above 22 |
| Rhythm | Regular | No change | Any change in rhythm or depth |

*Dental Emergencies*, First Edition. Edited by Mark Greenwood and Ian Corbett.
© 2012 Blackwell Publishing Ltd. Published 2012 by Blackwell Publishing Ltd.

# Appendix 3
# Warfarin Protocol

## Principles

Bleeding is easily treated using local measures so long as the international normalised ratio (INR) is known and patients with a level of 4 or less are being treated.

The risk of thromboembolism after withdrawal of warfarin therapy greatly outweighs the risk of bleeding.

A local anaesthetic containing a vasoconstrictor should be administered by infiltration or by intra-ligamentary injection wherever practical. Regional nerve blocks should be avoided if possible. If there is no alternative, however, local anaesthetic should be administered cautiously using an aspirating syringe.

After extraction, sockets should be gently packed with an absorbable haemostatic dressing, for example oxidised cellulose ('Surgicel®') or collagen sponge ('Haemocollagen'), then carefully sutured. Pressure should be applied by using a gauze pad that the patient bites down on for 15–30 minutes.

Patients should be given clear instructions on the management of the clot in the post-operative period and advised as shown in Table A3.1.

## Should the INR be measured before a dental procedure?

Yes. An INR must be measured not more than 24 hours before the proposed procedure. Patients will need either to coordinate their dental treatment with the next planned INR measurement (difficult) or have an extra INR measured within 24 hours of their planned dental procedure. If the INR is very stable, as judged from the patient's anticoagulation booklet, a period of 72 hours from the last INR test may be acceptable.

Patients taking warfarin with the following medical problems should be treated with additional caution as follows:

- Liver impairment and/or alcoholism
- Renal failure
- Thrombocytopaenia, haemophilia or other disorders of haemostasis
- Those currently receiving a course of cytotoxic medication or radiotherapy

*Dental Emergencies*, First Edition. Edited by Mark Greenwood and Ian Corbett.
© 2012 Blackwell Publishing Ltd. Published 2012 by Blackwell Publishing Ltd.

**Table A3.1**  Post-operative instructions for a warfarinised patient.

- To look after the initial clot by resting, while the local anaesthetic wears off and the clot forms (2–3 h).
- To avoid rinsing the mouth for 24 h.
- Not to suck hard or stick the tongue or any foreign object into the socket.
- To avoid hot liquids and hard foods for the rest of the day.
- Not to chew on the affected side for 3 days.
- If bleeding continues or restarts, to apply pressure over the socket using a folded clean handkerchief or gauze pad. Place the pad over the socket and bite firmly for 15–30 min. If bleeding does not stop, the dentist should be contacted, repacking and re-suturing of the socket may be required.
- Who to contact if they have excessive or prolonged post-operative bleeding.
- To avoid taking non-steroidal anti-inflammatory drugs immediately post-operatively.
- They may have been given a mouthwash (tranexamic acid). This should be held in the mouth over the operative site for up to 4 times daily.

## Are there any drug interactions that are relevant to this patient group?

- *Amoxicillin*: There are anecdotal reports that amoxicillin interacts with warfarin causing increased prothrombin time and/or bleeding but documented cases of interaction are relatively rare. Patients requiring a course of amoxicillin should be advised to be vigilant of any signs of increased bleeding.
- *Clindamycin*: It does not interact with warfarin.
- *Metronidazole*: (CAUTION) Metronidazole interacts with warfarin and should be avoided wherever possible. If it cannot be avoided, the warfarin dose may need to be reduced by a third to a half in consultation with the anticoagulant prescriber.
- *Erythromycin*: It interacts with warfarin unpredictably and only affects certain individuals. Patients should be advised to be vigilant for any signs of increased bleeding.
- *Non-steroidal anti-inflammatory drugs (NSAIDs)*: Avoid NSAIDs. Care should be taken when using NSAIDS in patients on anticoagulant therapy due to the increased risk of bleeding from the gastrointestinal tract.

## Oral surgery patients

### INR 4 or less

- Continue warfarin as normal. Local haemostatic measures should be employed post-operatively, that is oxidised cellulose pack and suturing of surgical site.

- An ID block can be given.
- The INR should be ideally checked on the day of surgery (see the preceding text).

### INR more than 4

Warfarin may need to be adjusted but should be done in consultation with the patient's physician. Some patients require other forms of anticoagulation if the warfarin is stopped. This would be managed on an in-patient basis.

If agreement to adjustment is obtained, the normal method would be to stop the warfarin 2 days before the planned procedure and restart it on the same evening of the day the procedure was undertaken.

## Restorative patients

Most procedures in restorative dentistry present no significant risk.

An interior dental block (IDB) can be done safely if the INR is 4 or less. Infiltration anaesthesia does not carry a need for a pre-operative INR check.

For gingival surgery, scaling or root surface debridement an INR should be checked first and the procedure only undertaken if the INR is 4 or less.

A summary of restorative procedures and INR guidance is given in Table A3.2.

**Table A3.2**  Management considerations in warfarinised patients requiring restorative dental procedures.

| Procedure | Test | Guidance |
|-----------|------|----------|
| Gingival surgery | Yes | For example, gingivectomy, flap surgery, implant surgery |
| Scaling and root surface debridement | Yes/No clinical decision | Most routine scaling will not require a test if the warfarin booklet show a consistent level of less than 3. A clinical judgement regarding bleeding risk should be made prior to taking the decision to test |
| Inferior dental block anaesthesia | Yes | Consider other routes of anaesthesia if possible, e.g. intra-ligamentary, mental block |
| All other restorative procedures | No | Includes preparations, matrix band placement, the use of retraction cord, endodontics, etc. |

# Checklist for patients taking warfarin who require dental treatment

## When arranging treatment

- Check that the treatment requires an INR to be carried out.
- Ensure sufficient appointment length arranged to maximise treatment possibilities.
- Have a look at the patient's warfarin record card to get an idea of the degree of anticoagulation and its stability.
- Ensure that there is sufficient time pre-treatment to get a blood sample and the result returned (may not be as critical if a clinical monitor is being used).

## On the day of treatment

- Check the INR.
- Verbal confirmation from the patient that they have complied with any changes to the warfarin treatment.
- Check that the patient fits into the categories outlined on the previous page.
- Remember to institute good local haemostatic measures.
- The use of tranexamic acid mouthwash, which acts as a local antifibrinolytic agent, may be made up on an individual basis by the hospital pharmacy.
- Avoid prescribing drugs that interact with warfarin.
- Ensure that the patient is given comprehensive post-operative instructions and that they have a point of contact should problems arise.

# Appendix 4

# Aspects Relating to Local Anaesthetics

Table A4.1   Classification of local anaesthetics.

| Amides | Esters |
| --- | --- |
| Lidocaine | Benzocaine |
| Prilocaine | Procaine |
| Mepivacaine | Tetracaine |
| Articaine | |
| Bupivacaine | |
| Ropivacaine | |

Table A4.2   Maximum doses for some commonly used local anaesthetics in dentistry.

| | |
| --- | --- |
| Lidocaine | 4.4 mg/kg |
| Articaine | 7.0 mg/kg |
| Mepivacaine | 4.4 mg/kg |
| Prilocaine | 6.0 mg/kg |

*Dental Emergencies*, First Edition. Edited by Mark Greenwood and Ian Corbett.
© 2012 Blackwell Publishing Ltd. Published 2012 by Blackwell Publishing Ltd.

# Appendix 5
# NICE Guidelines for the Removal of Wisdom Teeth

The National Institute for Health and Clinical Excellence (NICE) introduced guidelines in March 2000 to provide guidance for dentists and surgeons on deciding whether or not wisdom teeth should be removed. NICE concluded that there was no reliable research evidence to support a health benefit to patients from prophylactic removal of wisdom teeth and issued the following guidance:

(1) The routine practice of prophylactic removal of pathology-free impacted third molars should be discontinued in the National Health Service.
(2) Surgical removal of impacted third molars should be limited to those with evidence of pathology, such as the following:
   a. Unrestorable caries
   b. Fracture of tooth
   c. Non-treatable pulpal and/or periapical pathology
   d. Pathology of follicle including cyst/tumour
   e. Cellulitis or abscess formation
   f. Osteomyelitis
   g. Tooth/teeth impeding surgery, e.g. reconstructive jaw surgery, pre-prosthetic/implant surgery, orthognathic surgery, tooth involved within the field of tumour resection. Internal/external resorption of the tooth or adjacent teeth.
(3) Specific attention is drawn to plaque formation and pericoronitis. Plaque formation is a risk factor but is not itself an indication for surgery. The degree to which the severity of recurrence rate of pericoronitis should influence the decision for surgical removal of a third molar remains unclear. The evidence suggests that a first episode of pericoronitis, unless particularly severe, should not be considered an indication for surgery. Second or subsequent episodes should be considered as an appropriate indication for surgery.

*Dental Emergencies*, First Edition. Edited by Mark Greenwood and Ian Corbett.
© 2012 Blackwell Publishing Ltd. Published 2012 by Blackwell Publishing Ltd.

Each wisdom tooth should be assessed individually regarding the need for removal. It is good practice to clearly document the indication for removal of each tooth in the notes.

It is important to be aware that there are other indications for removal of impacted wisdom teeth that are not mentioned in the NICE guidelines. The Royal College of Surgeons guidelines, published in 1997 include the following as indications for removal:

- Restorative treatment (caries in adjacent tooth)
- Periodontal disease
- Orthodontic treatment
- Occupational (armed forces)
- Prophylactic removal for medical/surgical indications
- Donor transplantation.

# Appendix 6
# Protocol for Surgical Dental Treatment of Patients Taking Bisphosphonates

## Introduction and background

The use of bisphosphonates is associated with the production of osteonecrosis of the jaws (ONJ). ONJ is defined as exposure of the bone of the jaws that does not heal within 8 weeks after identification by a healthcare worker in a patient taking bisphosphonates. The condition may be asymptomatic or present with pain, soft-tissue swelling and loosening of teeth in addition to exposure of bone.

Bisphosphonates are inhibitors of osteoclastic activity and their presence in the body may last for years. These drugs are used in the management of the following:

- Malignancy:
  - To prevent hypercalcaemia
  - To reduce bone loss
- Osteoporosis
- Paget's disease of bone
- Osteogenesis imperfecta

When used in the management of malignancy the drugs are usually administered intravenously (IV). In the treatment of osteoporosis, the drug is normally taken orally. Although intravenous bisphosphonates may be used in the management of osteoporosis, the cumulative dose is lower than that used to manage the malignancy population. It is the intravenous route that is most commonly associated with the production of ONJ. The risk of ONJ in patients taking oral bisphosphonates is thought to be low but has been reported. Concomitant steroid therapy may increase the risk in the latter group.

It has been estimated that the percentage of patients receiving bisphosphonates for management of malignancy who develop ONF is between 4%

*Dental Emergencies*, First Edition. Edited by Mark Greenwood and Ian Corbett.
© 2012 Blackwell Publishing Ltd. Published 2012 by Blackwell Publishing Ltd.

and 10%. Around 60% of cases arise after tooth extraction or dento-alveolar surgery. The mandible is more susceptible than the maxilla.

In summary, it appears that the most at-risk group are patients receiving intravenous bisphosphonates during the management of malignancy.

### The bisphosphonate drugs

- Alendronic acid (Fosavance)
- Disodium etidronate (Didronel)
- Disodium pamidronate[a] (Aredia)
- Ibandronic acid[a] (Bondronat, Bonviva)
- Risedronate sodium (Actonel)
- Sodium clodronate[a] (Bonefos, Loron)
- Tiludronic acid (Skelid)
- Zoledronic acid[a] (Zometa)

[a]May be administered IV.

### Local risk factors for ONJ

The following are considered local risk factors for the production of ONJ:

- Poor oral hygiene
- Oral infection
- Dental extractions
- Bone manipulation
- Trauma from dentures
- Vasoconstrictors in local anaesthetics

## Management of patients taking bisphosphonates

There are currently no evidence-based protocols for the management of patients at risk of, or suffering from bisphosphonate-induced ONJ. Recommendations are based on expert opinion and can be considered under the headings of prevention, routine dental treatment of patients taking bisphosphonates and treating the patient with ONJ. The following recommendations should be followed when dealing with patients receiving intravenous bisphosphonate therapy; however, they should be considered in patients taking this group of drugs orally.

### Prevention

Prevention is key. Ideally, all patients about to receive intravenous bisphosphonate therapy should have a full dental assessment with necessary treatment prior to commencing therapy and all dental treatment completed.

It is thought that the incidence of ONJ is low within 6 months of the commencement of bisphosphonate therapy and thus patients who have just started this therapy should have a thorough dental assessment and treatment if this was not carried out prophylactically.

## Routine treatment of patients receiving bisphosphonates

The following are recommended in the routine dental management of patients receiving bisphosphonates:

- Maintenance of oral hygiene.
- Routine restorative dentistry should avoid soft tissue injury.
- Perform routine scalings but avoid soft tissue injury.
- Inspect and adjust removable prostheses for potential soft tissue injury.
- Treat dental infections aggressively but avoid surgery, if possible.
- Endodontics is preferable to extraction. Coronectomy with root canal therapy may be an option.
- Only grossly mobile teeth should be considered for extraction. An atraumatic technique is essential. Primary closure of wounds may be helpful. The use of prophylactic and post-operative antibiotics (preferably amoxicillin or clindamycin) should be used. Patients should be followed-up till healing is complete.

## Treatment of patients with bisphosphonate-induced ONJ

### Restorative dentistry
Routine restorative care should be provided under local anaesthesia. It is probably wise to use a vasoconstrictor-free solution.

### Periodontal treatment
Scaling can be performed but damage to soft tissue should be avoided.

### Endodontics
Teeth with pulpal involvement should be treated endodontically.

### Extractions
Only grossly mobile teeth should be considered for extraction. An atraumatic technique is essential. Primary closure of wounds may be helpful. The use of prophylactic and post-operative antibiotics (preferably amoxicillin or clindamycin) should be used. Chlorhexidine rinses should be advised pre- and post-operatively. Patients to be followed up until healing is complete.

### Implantology
Implants should generally be avoided in patients receiving bisphosphonates.

**Management of affected bone**

Surgery should be minimised and only sharp bony edges removed.

Chlorhexidine rinses should be used four times a day. Topical application of chlorhexidine gel may be helpful.

Antibiotics should be prescribed if there is evidence of infection around the exposed bone. Amoxicillin (500 mg four times a day initially followed by twice a day for maintenance) is useful. Clindamycin is the alternative if allergic to penicillin (150–300 mg four times daily) but limit to no more than 2-week course.

Antifungals may be required.

Dentures can be worn but must be adjusted to avoid soft tissue trauma and may be soft-lined.

## Further reading

American Association of Oral and Maxillofacial Surgeons. Position paper on bisphosphonate-related osteonecrosis of the jaw – 2009 update.

Cartsos VM, et al (2008) Bisphosphonate use and the risk of adverse jaw outcomes – a medical claims study of 714,217 people. *JADA* **139**, 23–30.

Grbic GT et al (2008) Incidence of osteonecrosis of the jaw in women with post-menopausal osteoporosis in the health outcomes and reduced incidence with zoledronic acid once yearly pivotal fracture trial. *JADA* **139**, 32–40.

# Appendix 7
# Common 'Recreational' Drugs

## Introduction

It is not uncommon in the dental emergency clinic to encounter patients who have a history of past or current recreational drug use. It is important that the dental practitioner has a basic understanding of the more common groups of drugs of abuse. Dental problems such as caries and periodontal disease are common among drug abusers. The combined effect of a poor diet, for example from carbohydrate additives to drugs and side effects from the abused drug such as a dry mouth as well as other factors are all implicated. This is important as it may impact on the treatment they receive or require. It is not possible to be totally exhaustive of all the drugs that the patients may be taking, but some of the more common ones are discussed in the following sections. A summary of the impact of some drugs of abuse on dentistry are given in Table A7.1.

Treatment is often sought at a late stage as the drug being abused may mask pain and discomfort caused by the oral disease.

General health issues need to be borne in mind in this group of patients. Cardiac and hepatic disease may result from the intravenous use of illicit drugs and sharing of needles increases the risk of viral infections. Illicit drugs may also interact with prescription medications, including those prescribed by dentists.

### Nicotine

Nicotine is the most widely used drug of abuse and its use is legal although it is discouraged for public health reasons. Nicotine causes raised blood pressure and will increase the rate of progression of cardiovascular disease. It is the chemicals that are taken along with nicotine in a cigarette that do most of the damage. Dental hospitals now have access to smoking cessation services, which are widely used.

It is particularly important that patients who present with oral mucosal lesions that have an etiology in smoking are referred appropriately for such counselling.

*Dental Emergencies*, First Edition. Edited by Mark Greenwood and Ian Corbett.
© 2012 Blackwell Publishing Ltd. Published 2012 by Blackwell Publishing Ltd.

**Table A7.1** The impact of drugs of abuse on dentistry.

| | Teeth | Oral mucosa | GA/ sedation | LA with adrenaline | Bleeding | Cardiac effects | HIV/ hepatitis | Drug interactions |
|---|---|---|---|---|---|---|---|---|
| Alcohol | + | + | + | | + | + | | + |
| Nicotine | + | + | + | | | | | |
| Cannabis | | + | + | + | | | | |
| Opioids | | | + | | + | + | + | + |
| CNS depressants | | + | + | | + | | | + |
| CNS stimulants | | + | + | + | + | + | + | + |
| Hallucinogens | | | | + | | | | + |
| Solvents | | | + | + | | + | | |
| Anabolic steroids/ performance enhancers | | | + | | + | + | + | + |

*Source:* From Greenwood M et al (2009) *Textbook of Human Disease in Dentistry.* Oxford: Wiley-Blackwell. Reproduced with permission from John Wiley & Sons Ltd. GA, general anaesthesia; LA, local anaesthesia; +, an interaction between the drug and the structure/function indicated.

**Table A7.2**  Number of units of alcohol in common drinks.

- A pint of ordinary strength lager – 2 units
- A pint of strong lager – 3 units
- A pint of ordinary bitter – 2 units
- A pint of best bitter – 3 units
- A pint of ordinary strength cider – 2 units
- A pint of strong cider – 3 units
- A 175 mL glass of red or white wine – around 2 units
- A pub measure of spirits – 1 unit
- An alcopop – around 1.5 units

## Alcohol

Alcohol is very widely consumed in many societies. The public health message with alcohol is different to nicotine in that up to certain levels of consumption it probably has beneficial effects. Alcohol abuse should be suspected if the patient smells of alcohol or has a marked tremor, which could be due to withdrawal. Attention should be paid to the time of the day, as many alcohol dependent patients will drink early in the morning to overcome symptoms of withdrawal.

The CAGE questionnaire is a useful screening tool that can be used to detect alcohol dependency. A negative CAGE response does not rule out alcohol abuse but a score of 2 or more is highly indicative of an alcohol problem. The CAGE questionnaire is given as follows:

C: Have you ever felt you should Cut down the amount you drink?
A: Are you Annoyed if people comment upon the amount you are drinking?
G: Do you ever feel Guilty about the amount you are drinking?
E: Have you ever had a drink early in the morning as an 'Eye-opener'?

Recommended maximum limits for males and females in terms of weekly alcohol consumption are 21 units and 14 units, respectively. The amount of alcohol contained in most common alcoholic drinks is given in the Table A7.2.

## Solvent abuse

The circumoral erythema known as 'glue-sniffers rash' may be seen in solvent abusers. Oral frostbite may be seen from the abuse of some aerosols.

Reduction in the dose of adrenaline-containing local anaesthetics is recommended in chronic solvent abusers as such agents can sensitise the myocardium to the actions of the catecholamine. As solvent abuse also increases the risk of convulsions, status epilepticus is a risk in this group of patients.

## Anabolic steroids and performance enhancing drugs

Anabolic steroids and performance enhancing drugs can precipitate excessive consumption of carbohydrates thereby increasing the incidence of dental caries. The systemic effects of adrenaline in local anaesthetics can be exacerbated by those performance-enhancing drugs that have a sympathomimetic action. As with many illicit drugs, anabolic steroids may interfere with blood clotting.

## Ecstasy

Ecstasy or 3,4-methylenedioxy-$n$-methlyamphetamine is a synthetic chemical. It is taken in tablet form and some also contain other psychoactive chemicals such as amphetamines (speed), LSD (acid) and caffeine as well as a number of other synthetic chemicals.

Ecstasy is as a stimulant. It increases brain activity and causes serotonin to be released from the brain. Serotonin is involved in the control of mood, emotions, sleep and pain perception. The latter is particularly important to the emergency dentist.

Short-term or immediate effects of ecstasy include increased heart rate as well as hypertension. The drug may cause xerostomia and raise body temperature – hence patients taking ecstasy tend to run the risk of dehydration and often tend to overcompensate by drinking large quantities of fluid.

Patients taking ecstasy in large quantities may suffer from anxiety and panic attacks and as the drug wears off, depression may develop.

It is not thought that taking ecstasy generally leads to addiction. A degree of tolerance to the drug builds up and therefore users tend to take more and more of the drug to have the same effect. It is possible for patients to become psychologically dependent on the drug.

## Cannabis

Cannabis is a drug that is produced from a plant related to nettles and hops. Used in its recreational form, the drug takes many forms such as herbal, resin, powder and oil. Patients will refer to cannabis by some of its slang terms such as weed, pot, grass and hash. It is usually rolled into the form of a cigarette that is referred to as a 'joint'. Tetrahydrocannabinol is the main active ingredient. The drug acts as a mild sedative. Cannabis can also have mild hallucinogenic effects and reduces inhibitions.

There is evidence that cannabis can be used therapeutically in a wide variety of disorders, particularly multiple sclerosis but also for migraine, headaches, Parkinson's disease, Alzheimer's disease and others.

Cannabis can be associated with deleterious health effects however. In teenagers, it can affect psychological development and ability to concentrate. There may be effects on the heart including increased heart rate and blood pressure. Attempts to withdraw from the drug can lead to cravings, mood changes and agitation.

## Amphetamines

Amphetamines have been prescribed therapeutically for several disorders. Due to their addictive potential, they have largely fallen out of use for therapeutic applications in most cases and are now more widely used as illicit drugs. The drug usually comes in powder or tablet form and may be referred to by the slang term as 'speed' or 'uppers'.

One form of amphetamines (also known as crystal meth) is a similar but more powerful type of the drug. Users of amphetamines will use the powder by snorting into the nose or rubbing it into the gums. Tablets are sometimes swallowed. It can be used by injection.

Amphetamines increase levels of dopamine and noradrenaline in the brain which potentiates the stimulant effects. Large amounts can lead to significant psychological problems, including a sense of panic and paranoia. Palpitations, risk of arrhythmia and myocardial infarction are significant risks as are low blood pressure, nausea, headache and tremor.

Users of amphetamines can become chronically tired and are particularly vulnerable to infections due to their 'run down' state. Depression may also occur along with aggression and psychosis.

## Cocaine

Cocaine is manufactured from the leaves of a South American shrub. It is a stimulant drug that is highly addictive. It is usually taken as a fine white powder snorted into the nose. It can also be injected.

Long-term users of cocaine can develop anxiety and panic attacks. Physical effects include myocardial infarction, stroke, respiratory problems and seizures.

One of the characteristic features of cocaine use is that tolerance can develop quite rapidly. Effects of cocaine are very short-lived and it does not have the same type and degree of physical withdrawal effects as other drugs.

The vasoconstrictor action of cocaine can lead to ischaemia, with subsequent tissue loss. Patients who use the drug by rubbing onto the oral mucosa may lead to loss of gingivae and alveolar bone. Similarly, dental caries may occur as a result of the drug being bulked out with carbohydrates.

## Heroin

Heroin is derived from opium. Heroin (diamorphine) is used medically, particularly for analgesia in myocardial infarction patients as well as analgesia in patients who have severe pain. Users of heroin feel euphoric, warm and relaxed. Pupils will be markedly constricted and speech may become slurred. Heroin is a drug that is highly addictive and tolerance builds up quickly. The drug is short acting so several 'fixes' may be needed in the same day. This is largely to avoid withdrawal symptoms such as shivers and sweats, muscle cramps and watering eyes and nose.

The main risks from heroin use is the risk of developing HIV infection or hepatitis from using contaminated needles, as well as physical damage to veins used for injection leading to the development of thrombosis and possible abscesses. Damage to the lungs can occur with a condition developing resembling asthma.

Heroin interacts with some drugs that dentists may prescribe. For example, the absorption of paracetamol and orally administered diazepam delayed and reduced as a result of delayed gastric emptying.

## Lysergic acid diethylamide

LSD (lysergic acid diethylamide) is a systemic chemical manufactured from a fungus that grows on rye. It is one of the most powerful known hallucinogens. It may work by blocking serotonin in the brain and activating dopamine. The drug stimulates the sympathetic nervous system. It is commonly known as 'acid'. Experience of using LSD, commonly referred to as a 'trip', can be very unpredictable. It can be a very pleasant experience but some users may find a trip disturbing which can cause significant psychological damage. On taking LSD, the trip does not start straight away but can take anything from 20 minutes to a couple of hours. The drug is not physically addictive but tolerance may develop. Psychological addiction may develop however.

## Mephedrone and naphyrone

Mephedrone and naphyrone are plant derived. These drugs can produce mild euphoria and reduce appetite. Mephedrone is a yellow powder whereas naphyrone is a white crystalline powder. Both can be snorted as well as taken by other routes.

The drugs can have physical as well as psychological adverse effects. The main physical effects are on the cardiovascular system leading to tachycardia. Arterial constriction can lead to peripheral cyanosis.

## Methadone

Methadone is a synthetic substance that is prescribed for patients who are addicted to heroin. It has similar but less marked effects. It is potentially addictive but less so than heroin. It is an effective analgesic and is often used to treat patients therapeutically. If taken in large amounts it produces side effects that are similar to those of heroin. Though methadone is addictive in its own right death rates are much less than those from heroin as a result of the close supervision of patients taking this drug.

Serum methadone levels are reduced when carbamazepine is prescribed. The effects of tricyclic antidepressants are increased in patients taking methadone.

## Analgesics

Analgesics such as aspirin, paracetamol and ibuprofen are not addictive. The person may become physically dependent on them however, in order to be able to carry out activities of daily living or to control their pain. They will not, however, become psychologically dependent in the strict sense of the term.

There is a small risk of addiction developing to some of the codeine containing compound analgesics. Codeine is an opiate and although its dose is small in such preparations it can still induce a feeling of general well-being, or sedation. As a result of this addiction can occur and a person may suffer withdrawal symptoms when they try to stop taking such drugs.

It is important for the dental practitioner to be wary of the patient who attends the clinic requesting a particular type of analgesia. It must be borne in mind that the patient may have a genuine reason for asking for this particular type of medication in that it has helped them in the past. Patients specifically requesting codeine containing preparations, however, should be treated with caution.

## Tranquilisers

The main group of drugs to which patients may become addicted are the benzodiazepine drugs such as diazepam and temazepam. They enhance the effect of gamma amino butyric acid (GABA). This depresses the central nervous system and leads to relaxation and sedation. Drugs such as zopiclone (Z drugs) pose a lower risk but also act on GABA receptors and in general are best not used long-term.

Tolerance can quickly develop to the benzodiazepine drugs. Therefore, it is important that they are not used long-term as it can be very difficult to wean patients off them.

## Conclusion

Dental practitioners should have a working knowledge of the main groups of drugs to which their patients may become addicted or develop dependence or tolerance.

# Index

*Dental Emergencies*, First Edition. Edited by Mark Greenwood and Ian Corbett.
© 2012 Blackwell Publishing Ltd. Published 2012 by Blackwell Publishing Ltd.

Printed and bound by CPI Group (UK) Ltd, Croydon, CR0 4YY

27/10/2024

14580144-0004